Understanding Dengue Fever

A Comprehensive Guide to Managing and Avoiding Dengue Infections

Brenda F. Dozier

Gratitude

Dear Readers,

We express our heartfelt gratitude to every one of you for choosing to invest your time and resources in Understanding Dengue Fever: A Comprehensive Guide to Managing and Avoiding Dengue Infections. Your decision to read this book is a testimonial to your commitment to bettering your awareness of a vital global health issue and contributing to a healthier, more educated world.

This book was written with the highest attention to delivering accurate, thorough, and accessible information about dengue fever. We acknowledge the importance of arming individuals, communities, and healthcare professionals with the knowledge needed to tackle this disease effectively. Your interaction with this information not only aids in your learning but also enhances the community effort to address and reduce the impact of dengue fever worldwide.

We are genuinely appreciative of your willingness to educate yourself about dengue fever, its spread, symptoms, and prevention techniques. Your proactive stance plays a significant part in the broader fight against this prevalent sickness. Every reader who becomes better informed about dengue helps to a ripple effect, increasing awareness and developing a more watchful and responsive global community.

Our warmest appreciation goes out to the medical experts, researchers, and public health advocates who have committed their lives to the study and control of dengue fever. Your tireless work and important contributions have set the foundation for this book, giving the critical insights and data that make full knowledge possible.

We also like to acknowledge the individuals and families who have been afflicted by dengue disease. Your experiences and tales are a poignant reminder of why continued education, research, and worldwide collaboration are vital. This book is, in part, a monument to your resilience and a call to action to prevent others from facing similar experiences.

To every reader, thank you for being part of this journey towards improved knowledge and health security. Your chase of understanding and your devotion to health literacy are laudable. We hope that this book gives you the understanding and methods necessary to protect yourself and your loved ones against dengue fever and inspires you to spread this critical information throughout your community.

With sincere gratitude,

[Brenda F. Dozier]

Table of Contents

Introduction

It is estimated that millions of individuals worldwide are at risk of contracting dengue fever, a viral infection transmitted by mosquitoes. Understanding and effectively managing dengue fever remains a formidable obstacle for many people, although it is one of the most prevalent and quickly spreading infections. Since the disease is extremely complicated and has the potential to have a devastating impact, people, families, and communities must be well-informed and prepared.
To successfully navigate the complex world of dengue fever, you will find that this book, "Understanding Dengue Fever: A Comprehensive Guide to Managing and Avoiding Dengue Infections," is an indispensable resource.

Imagine yourself waking up one morning with a high fever, horrible headaches, and intense agony in your joints and muscles. Dengue fever can cause its sufferers to experience a wide range of debilitating symptoms, some of which are listed below, for example. A diagnosis of dengue fever can be extremely overwhelming due to the feelings of uncertainty, anxiety, and helplessness that accompany it. However, with the correct knowledge and tactics, you can effectively manage the disease and protect yourself and your loved ones from its grasp.

Through the publication of this book, we hope to provide you with the most precise, up-to-date, and applicable information currently accessible. We dig into the history and spread of dengue, presenting insights into its transmission through the famed Aedes mosquitoes. Through this course, you will acquire a comprehensive grasp of the various varieties of dengue viruses, how they function, and the symptoms that they give rise to. With this information, you will be able to spot the symptoms at an earlier stage and seek medical assistance at the appropriate time.

But knowing about dengue fever is just the beginning. This guide goes further, exploring complete treatment and management alternatives. From medical treatments to home care remedies, we provide you with a holistic approach to easing the symptoms and speeding up recovery. The importance of water and nutrition, frequently underestimated, is addressed to ensure you have all the skills essential for efficient treatment.

Prevention is supreme in the fight against dengue disease. We offer extensive plans for mosquito control, personal safety, and environmental management. Whether you reside in a high-risk location or plan to go to one, this book empowers you with practical guidance to limit your risk of infection. The collective effort of communities and the role of public health programs are also emphasized, underscoring that we all have a part to play in combating this disease.

In a world where the dengue virus continues to cost lives and devastate communities, this book is not just a guide; it is a lifeline. By understanding the global impact and the difficulty of eliminating dengue, you will realize the urgency and significance of remaining informed. We also look to the future, investigating exciting research and breakthroughs in dengue prevention and treatment.

Our journey through this book is not only academic; it is extremely personal. We share stories and ideas from dengue survivors, delivering a human touch that connects with empathy and optimism. These experiences remind us that while dengue disease can be a powerful foe, resilience, and knowledge can triumph.

Understanding Dengue Fever: A Comprehensive Guide to Managing and Avoiding Dengue Infections" is more than a book; it is your friend in the fight against dengue. Let this guide be your beacon of knowledge, empowering you to take charge and make informed decisions. Together, we can outsmart dengue fever and pave the way for healthier, safer lives.

Overview of dengue fever

Dengue fever is a mosquito-borne virus-related disease caused by the dengue virus, which is transferred to humans through the bite of an infected Aedes mosquito, particularly Aedes aegypti. This mosquito species is very efficient at spreading the virus due to its affection for human blood and its habit of staying near people. Aedes mosquitoes are most active during the day, with peak biting hours in the early morning and late afternoon.

The dengue virus belongs to the Flavivirus genus and has four unique serotypes: DENV-1, DENV-2, DENV-3, and DENV-4. Infection with one serotype affords permanent immunity against that specific serotype but provides only partial and transitory immunity against the others. Subsequent infections with various serotypes raise the risk of developing severe dengue, regularly known as dengue hemorrhagic fever (DHF) or dengue shock syndrome (DSS).

The symptoms of dengue fever normally develop 4-10 days after the mosquito bite and include high fever, severe headache, pain behind the eyes, joint and muscular pain, rash, and moderate bleeding (such as nose or gum bleeding and easy bruising). These symptoms can range from moderate to severe, and in some circumstances, they can be life-threatening. Severe dengue is characterized by plasma leakage, fluid accumulation, respiratory difficulty, severe bleeding, and organ damage.

Early identification and appropriate medical care are critical to lower the risk of complications and mortality. There is no specific antiviral treatment for dengue, and management generally focuses on treating symptoms and preserving the patient's fluid balance. Supportive care, including rehydration and pain medication, is required, particularly for severe instances.

Historical Context and Global Impact

Dengue fever has a lengthy history, with allusions to dengue-like disorders dating back to ancient China over 2,000 years ago. However, the earliest recognized dengue outbreaks occurred in the late 18th century in Asia, Africa, and North America. The term "dengue" is believed to have arisen from the Swahili phrase "Ka-dinga pepo," denoting a sudden cramp-like seizure induced by an evil spirit. Spanish colonists later changed the phrase to "dengue."

The global spread of dengue fever intensified in the 20th century due to urbanization, increasing travel, and inadequate mosquito control efforts. During World War II, army movements and supply lines aided the spread of Aedes mosquitoes and the dengue virus across Southeast Asia and the Pacific. In the ensuing decades, dengue fever emerged as a substantial public health hazard in many tropical and subtropical locations.

The 1950s heralded the onset of serious dengue epidemics, commencing in the Philippines and Thailand. These outbreaks emphasized the potential severity of the disease and its capacity to inflict severe morbidity and mortality. By the late 20th century, dengue fever had become endemic in over 100 countries, with the Americas, Southeast Asia, and the Western Pacific areas most impacted.

In recent years, the global incidence of dengue has climbed considerably. According to the World Health Organization (WHO), the number of reported cases has increased more than 30-fold over the past 50 years. This spike can be ascribed to various factors, including population expansion, urbanization, international travel, climate change, and poor vector control efforts. Today, an estimated 390 million dengue infections occur annually, with around 96 million resulting in clinical symptoms.

Importance of Understanding and Managing Dengue Infections

Understanding and managing dengue infections is of critical importance due to the severe health, economic, and societal repercussions of the disease. Dengue fever affects millions of individuals each year, causing extensive disease, economic burden, and loss of productivity. The disease disproportionately affects low- and middle-income nations, where healthcare resources may be limited, and public health infrastructure may be weak.

One of the key issues in managing dengue is the lack of effective antiviral medicines. Currently, there is no cure for dengue fever, and therapy generally focuses on treating symptoms and providing supportive care. This makes early identification and appropriate medical intervention vital to minimize complications and reduce mortality. Health practitioners must be well-trained to detect the signs and symptoms of dengue and differentiate it from other febrile infections.

Preventing dengue infections relies mainly on managing the mosquito vectors that carry the virus. Effective vector management tactics include reducing breeding areas, employing pesticides, and promoting the use of mosquito repellents and protective apparel. Community participation and education are key components of these activities, as individuals and communities play a vital role in lowering mosquito populations and preventing mosquito bites.

Vaccination also has promise in the fight against dengue. The first dengue vaccine, Dengvaxia, was approved for use in several countries in 2015. However, its usage is limited to persons who have already been infected with dengue, as it may raise the risk of severe dengue in those who are dengue-naive. Ongoing research and development efforts are focused on generating more effective and broadly applicable vaccinations to protect populations at risk.

The economic burden of dengue fever is enormous. The expenditures involved with medical treatment, hospitalization, and missed productivity can strain healthcare systems and economies, particularly in endemic locations. Investing in prevention and control efforts can lessen these cost burdens and enhance overall public health outcomes.

Furthermore, the societal impact of dengue cannot be neglected. The disease affects individuals of all ages, but children are more prone to severe dengue and its sequelae. The emotional and psychological toll on patients and their families is enormous, as they cope with the worry and uncertainty of the condition. Public health campaigns and educational programs can assist raise awareness, eliminate stigma, and promote early detection and treatment.

Global Impact and Epidemiology

Dengue fever is a global health hazard, with its impact felt most acutely in tropical and subtropical countries. The illness is endemic in over 100 countries, with the biggest burden in the Americas, Southeast Asia, and the Western Pacific. However, dengue cases have also been reported in Africa, the Eastern Mediterranean, and even portions of Europe, indicating the extensive reach of the disease.

The epidemiology of dengue fever is impacted by several factors, including climate, urbanization, and human behavior. Aedes mosquitoes flourish in warm, humid conditions, making tropical and subtropical countries highly prone to dengue outbreaks. Climate change is projected to expand the geographic range of these insects, potentially increasing the number of humans at risk for dengue infection.

Urbanization has an impact on the spread of dengue. Rapid population expansion and unplanned urban development create excellent circumstances for mosquito breeding. Poor sanitation, inadequate waste management, and the proliferation of discarded containers that can store water contribute to the increase in mosquito populations. In densely populated metropolitan settings, the close contact of individuals increases the transmission of the virus.

International travel and trade have also contributed to this global spread of dengue. Infected travelers can bring the virus to new places, leading to local transmission when Aedes mosquitoes are present. This pattern has been documented in previous epidemics in non-endemic locations, underlining the necessity of surveillance and preventive actions for visitors.

The burden of dengue is not uniformly distributed, with certain nations and regions seeing higher rates of infection and more severe outbreaks. For example, throughout the Americas, dengue prevalence has climbed considerably over the past several decades, with Brazil accounting for a significant number of cases. In Southeast Asia, nations such as Thailand, Indonesia, and the Philippines record significant numbers of dengue cases annually. The Western Pacific area, comprising nations like Vietnam and Malaysia, also has substantial hurdles in managing dengue.

The impact of dengue spreads beyond human health, influencing economies and healthcare systems. The cost of dengue is enormous, comprising direct medical bills, vector control measures, and lost productivity. In endemic nations, dengue outbreaks can overwhelm healthcare institutions, leading to resource shortages and strained medical services. The economic impact is particularly onerous for low- and middle-income countries, where resources may already be constrained.

Efforts to eradicate dengue involve a diverse approach, involving governments, healthcare providers, researchers, and communities. Surveillance and monitoring are vital for early detection and response to outbreaks. Integrated vector management tactics, integrating chemical, biological, and environmental control measures, can help reduce mosquito populations and prevent transmission. Public education initiatives are vital for raising awareness and supporting preventive practices.

Research and innovation are essential components of the global response to dengue. Advances in diagnostic techniques, therapy choices, and vaccine development offer hope for more effective management and prevention of the condition. Collaboration between international organizations, governments, and the business sector may drive progress and guarantee that the benefits of new technology and initiatives reach those most in need.

Chapter 1

Understanding Dengue Fever

Dengue fever is a mosquito-borne viral disease that has become a substantial public health concern in many parts of the world. This illness is caused by the dengue virus, which is transmitted to people predominantly by the Aedes aegypti mosquito. Dengue fever appears with a wide spectrum of symptoms, from mild febrile illness to severe and life-threatening diseases. The disease has undergone a rapid surge in occurrence over recent decades, making it vital to understand its biology, history, and transmission pathways.

What is Dengue Fever?

Dengue fever is an acute viral infection characterized by quick onset of high fever, severe headache, pain behind the eyes, joint and muscle pain, rash, and moderate bleeding (such as nose or gum bleeding and easy bruising). The disease is caused by the dengue virus, which belongs to the Flavivirus genus. There are four separates but closely related, serotypes of the virus: DENV-1, DENV-2, DENV-3, and DENV-4. Infection with one serotype offers lifetime immunity to that specific serotype but only partial and transitory immunity to the other serotypes.

The clinical appearance of dengue might vary greatly. In many circumstances, individuals may develop moderate or asymptomatic illnesses. However, in severe cases, dengue fever can develop into dengue hemorrhagic fever (DHF) or dengue shock syndrome (DSS), all of which are potentially lethal. DHF is characterized by high fever, damage to blood and lymph arteries, bleeding from the nose and mouth, enlarged liver, and, in extreme cases, circulatory failure. DSS is a critical moment where a sudden drop in blood pressure can lead to shock and mortality if not properly treated.

History and Global Prevalence of Dengue

The history of dengue fever extends back hundreds of years, with records of dengue-like disorders in ancient Chinese medical writings as early as 992 AD. The first well-documented outbreak happened in the 1780s concurrently throughout Asia, Africa, and North America. However, it was not until the early 20th century that dengue fever was separated from other febrile disorders by virological and epidemiological investigations.

The global spread of dengue fever surged post-World War II due to increasing travel, urbanization, and poor mosquito control efforts. By the 1950s and 1960s, dengue had become endemic in many tropical and subtropical locations. Major outbreaks were documented in Southeast Asia and the Western Pacific, demonstrating the terrible impact of the disease.

In the later half of the 20th century and into the 21st century, the incidence of dengue fever has continued to climb substantially. According to the World Health Organization (WHO), dengue is currently widespread in over 100 countries, with an estimated 390 million dengue illnesses occurring each year. Approximately 96 million of these infections result in clinical signs of the disease. The regions most affected include Southeast Asia, the Western Pacific, the Americas, and parts of Africa. The growing prevalence of dengue fever is ascribed to causes such as population growth, urbanization, increased travel, climate change, and inefficient vector control efforts.

Types of Dengue Viruses and Their Characteristics

The dengue virus has four unique serotypes: DENV-1, DENV-2, DENV-3, and DENV-4. These serotypes are genetically similar but differ enough to induce diverse immunological responses. Infection with one serotype often offers lifelong immunity to that serotype but does not provide permanent immunity to the other three serotypes. This characteristic of partial immunity is crucial because it means that individuals can be infected with dengue numerous times during their lives, each time by a different serotype.

DENV-1: This serotype is generally associated with more conventional symptoms of dengue fever. It is one of the most ubiquitous serotypes and has been responsible for several large outbreaks globally. DENV-1 infections can lead to severe disease, especially in places where the population has had limited previous exposure to the virus.

DENV-2: This serotype is frequently connected to more severe types of dengue, including DHF and DSS. DENV-2 has been involved with multiple serious outbreaks, mainly in Southeast Asia and the Americas. Studies have revealed that DENV-2 may have a higher potential to produce severe disease compared to the other serotypes.

DENV-3: DENV-3 is renowned for its relationship with plain dengue outbreaks. This serotype has created considerable public health concerns in regions such as Southeast Asia, the Americas, and the Western Pacific. Like DENV-2, DENV-3 can lead to severe illness, especially in populations with limited immunity to this serotype.

DENV-4: While DENV-4 is often less virulent compared to DENV-2 and DENV-3, it still offers a substantial hazard in dengue-endemic areas. DENV-4 has produced epidemics in locations like as Southeast Asia and the Pacific Islands. Its presence adds to the complex epidemiology of dengue, where different serotypes can co-circulate and lead to sequential infections.

The interaction between different dengue serotypes has a significant role in the epidemiology and clinical presentation of the disease. Secondary infection with a different serotype raises the likelihood of severe disease due to a mechanism known as antibody-dependent enhancement (ADE). During a subsequent infection, non-neutralizing antibodies from the first infection may enhance the entry of the virus into host cells, leading to increased viral replication and a heightened immunological response. This process is believed to contribute to the severe symptoms of dengue, such as DHF and DSS.

Transmission of Dengue Virus (Mosquito Vector)

The principal mechanism of transmission of the dengue virus is through the bite of infected female Aedes mosquitoes, notably Aedes aegypti and Aedes albopictus. These mosquitoes are highly adapted to urban areas and have a strong affinity for feeding on human blood, making them efficient vectors for the dengue virus.

Aedes aegypti: Aedes aegypti is the primary vector of dengue virus. This mosquito species flourishes in urban and suburban environments, where it breeds in artificial containers such as abandoned tires, flower pots, water storage containers, and other items that may store water. Aedes aegypti mosquitoes are most active during the day, with peak biting hours in the early morning and late afternoon. They prefer to rest indoors, frequently in dark, cool spaces such as closets and beneath furniture, making them difficult to find and control.

Aedes albopictus: Also known as the Asian tiger mosquito, Aedes albopictus is a secondary vector of dengue virus. It is a very adaptable species that can survive in both urban and rural habitats. Aedes albopictus is less anthropophilic (preferring human blood) than Aedes aegypti, yet it is also active during the day. This mosquito species is capable of breeding in a wide range of natural and artificial containers, including tree holes, bamboo stumps, and discarded containers. Its capacity to thrive in varied settings and its aggressive biting habits contribute to its role in dengue transmission.

The transmission cycle of the dengue virus begins when a female Aedes mosquito bites an infected person and ingests the virus along with the blood meal. The virus then replicates in the mosquito's midgut and travels to other tissues, including the salivary glands. After an extrinsic incubation period of typically 8-12 days, the mosquito becomes infectious and can transfer the virus to another human by its bite.

Humans are the principal reservoir of dengue virus, meaning that the virus circulates within the human population and relies on human hosts for its transmission cycle. However, there is evidence that certain species of monkeys in specific places may also function as reservoirs for the virus.

The transmission dynamics of dengue are determined by various factors, including the density and dispersion of Aedes mosquitoes, the level of virus circulation in the human population, and environmental conditions. Warm temperatures and high humidity are conducive to mosquito breeding and viral replication, leading to enhanced transmission during the rainy season in many tropical and subtropical countries.

Vector control is an significant component of dengue prevention and control techniques. Reducing the population of Aedes mosquitoes and restricting their interaction with humans can dramatically minimize the risk of dengue transmission. Effective vector control measures include:

Eliminating Breeding Sites: Removing or frequently cleaning objects that can collect water, such as flower pots, abandoned tires, and water storage tanks, will reduce mosquito breeding habitats.

Insecticide Use: Applying insecticides to kill adult mosquitoes and larvae can help manage mosquito populations. This involves indoor residual spraying and space spraying (fogging) in locations with high mosquito concentrations.

Personal Protection: utilizing mosquito repellents, wearing long-sleeved clothing, and utilizing mosquito netting helps lower the risk of mosquito bites. Screening windows and doors can also help keep mosquitoes out of residential rooms.

Community Engagement: Engaging communities in vector control activities is vital for ongoing success. Public education efforts can raise awareness about the necessity of reducing breeding grounds and preventing mosquito bites.

In recent years, innovative approaches to vector control have been developed and used in several domains. These include the introduction of genetically modified mosquitoes that are sterile or carry a bacterium (Wolbachia) that decreases the mosquito's capacity to transmit the virus. These technologies offer intriguing new weapons in the fight against dengue but require rigorous research and monitoring to assess their efficiency and potential ecological consequences.

Understanding the biology and behavior of Aedes mosquitoes and the processes of dengue virus transmission is critical for designing effective preventative and control techniques. By lowering mosquito populations and restricting human exposure to mosquito bites, we can considerably reduce the incidence of dengue fever and its accompanying health and economic consequences.

Different Serotypes and Their Implications

The occurrence of four unique serotypes of the dengue virus has substantial implications for the epidemiology, clinical presentation, and therapy of dengue fever. One of the most significant implications is secondary infection, where a person previously infected with one serotype is later infected with a different serotype. This scenario can develop into a more severe disease due to a mechanism known as antibody-dependent enhancement (ADE).

During a subsequent infection, non-neutralizing antibodies from the first infection might accelerate the entry of the virus into host cells, leading to enhanced viral replication and a more robust immune response. This heightened immune reaction is likely to contribute to the development of severe types of dengue, such as DHF and DSS. Therefore, individuals who have undergone a first dengue infection are at greater risk of severe disease if they are subsequently infected with a different serotype.

The distribution of dengue serotypes varies geographically and temporally, with distinct serotypes predominating in different regions and seasons. Co-circulation of many serotypes is frequent in many dengue-endemic locations, complicating efforts to manage the disease and anticipate outbreaks. The shifting dominance of serotypes can lead to recurrent epidemics, as populations with insufficient immunity to the newly dominant serotype become susceptible.

Effective dengue preventive and control methods must account for the range of serotypes and the risk of severe disease associated with secondary infections. Surveillance programs that monitor circulating serotypes and detect changes in their distribution are vital for guiding public health initiatives and immunization tactics.

Lifecycle within the Mosquito Vector

The lifetime of the dengue virus within the mosquito vector, predominantly Aedes aegypti, contains several important stages. Understanding this lifetime is vital for establishing effective vector control techniques and halting the propagation of the virus.

Ingestion: The lifecycle begins when a female Aedes mosquito bites an infected human and ingests blood containing the dengue virus. The virus penetrates the mosquito's midgut, where it encounters digestive enzymes and begins to multiply.

Midgut Infection: The virus infects the epithelial cells of the midgut, replicating and creating new viral particles. This step is essential, as not all mosquitoes that swallow the virus will become infected. The efficacy of midgut infection can vary based on factors such as the mosquito's genetic composition and the viral load in the blood meal.

Dissemination: After successful replication in the midgut, the virus travels to other tissues within the mosquito, including the hemocoel (the mosquito's body cavity) and the salivary glands. The dissemination phase is necessary for the mosquito to become capable of spreading the virus to people.

Salivary Gland Infection: The virus must infect the salivary glands to be transferred to a new human host. Once the salivary glands are infected, the mosquito becomes infectious and can transfer the virus through its saliva when it bites another person.

Transmission: The extrinsic incubation period, which is the time from when the mosquito ingests the virus to when it may spread the virus, generally lasts 8-12 days. During this stage, the virus completes its reproduction and spread activities within the mosquito. Once the mosquito is contagious, it can transmit the virus to humans for the balance of its life, which can last many weeks.

Understanding the lifecycle of the dengue virus within Aedes mosquitoes shows the need to manage mosquito populations and minimize mosquito bites to limit the transmission of dengue illness.

Transmission via Aedes aegypti Mosquitoes

Aedes aegypti is the principal vector responsible for delivering the dengue virus to humans. This mosquito species is highly adaptable to urban areas and has a strong predilection for human blood. Several properties of Aedes aegypti contribute to its efficiency as a dengue vector.

Breeding Habits: Aedes aegypti mosquitoes reproduce in artificial containers that hold water, such as flower pots, abandoned tires, water storage tanks, and other items typically encountered in urban settings. These mosquitoes deposit their eggs in clean, standing water, and their eggs may withstand desiccation for several months, making them resilient to dry conditions.

Feeding Behavior: Aedes aegypti is an hostile daylight biter, with peak feeding hours in the early morning and late afternoon. These mosquitoes are drawn to human scent, body heat, and carbon dioxide, and they prefer to feed indoors, generally resting in dark, chilly regions such as closets and beneath furniture.

Host Preference: Aedes aegypti mosquitoes display a high preference for human blood over animal blood. This inclination enhances the possibility of virus transmission, as the mosquitoes commonly feed on several humans during their lifecycle, potentially spreading the virus from one sick person to another.

Flying Range: Aedes aegypti mosquitoes have a relatively restricted flying range, often less than 200 meters from their spawning locations. This narrow range means that localized mosquito control efforts, such as eliminating nesting areas and employing insecticides, can be effective in lowering the mosquito population and interrupting transmission.

Clinical Manifestations: From Mild Dengue Fever to Severe Forms

Dengue fever manifests with a variety of clinical symptoms, ranging from mild febrile sickness to severe and life-threatening diseases. The severity of the disease can vary greatly based on factors such as the patient's age, immunological condition, and whether they have been previously infected with a different dengue serotype.

Moderate Dengue Fever: The majority of dengue infections result in moderate disease, characterized by quick onset of high fever, severe headache, pain behind the eyes, joint and muscular pain, rash, and modest bleeding symptoms such as nose or gum bleeding and easy bruising. The fever normally lasts 2-7 days and is sometimes referred to as "breakbone fever" due to the acute joint and muscular pain experienced by patients. Most patients with moderate dengue recover totally within a few weeks, although they may endure persistent lethargy and weakness.

Dengue Hemorrhagic Fever (DHF): DHF is a severe form of dengue characterized by increased vascular permeability, plasma leakage, and bleeding tendencies. DHF is divided into four degrees of severity (I-IV), with grades III and IV considered the most severe. Symptoms of DHF include continuous high fever, severe abdominal discomfort, vomiting, bleeding from the nose, gums, or under the skin, and difficulty breathing. Plasma leakage can lead to fluid accumulation in bodily cavities, causing respiratory difficulty and organ damage. Timely medical intervention is vital to control DHF and prevent progression to dengue shock syndrome.

Dengue Shock Syndrome (DSS): DSS is the most severe type of dengue and occurs when plasma leakage leads to a significant drop in blood pressure and circulatory failure. Patients with DSS may present with symptoms of shock, such as cold, clammy skin, fast pulse, and altered mental status. DSS can be fatal if not promptly treated with fluid resuscitation and supportive treatment. Early detection and active care of DSS are critical to enhance patient outcomes and reduce death.

Warning signals: Dengue patients may exhibit warning signals signaling the progression to severe disease, particularly around the period of defervescence (when the fever starts to diminish). These warning indications include severe abdominal discomfort, frequent vomiting, fast breathing, bleeding gums, exhaustion, restlessness, and hepatomegaly (enlarged liver). The existence of these warning symptoms necessitates close monitoring and medical examination to prevent the development of severe dengue.

Diagnosis and Management: The diagnosis of dengue fever is mostly based on clinical presentation and laboratory investigations. Early diagnosis is critical for optimal care and to distinguish dengue from other febrile diseases. Laboratory techniques such as reverse transcription-polymerase chain reaction (RT-PCR), enzyme-linked immunosorbent assay (ELISA), and rapid diagnostic tests (RDTs) can detect the presence of the dengue virus or particular antibodies.

There is no specific antiviral medication for dengue fever, and management is mostly supportive. For moderate dengue, patients are advised to relax, keep appropriate hydration, and use acetaminophen for pain alleviation. Non-steroidal anti-inflammatory medicines (NSAIDs) such as ibuprofen and aspirin should be avoided due to the risk of bleeding.

Patients with DHF and DSS require hospitalization for thorough monitoring and intensive management. Intravenous fluid treatment is needed to maintain blood volume and prevent shock. The fluid replacement method should be carefully calibrated to minimize fluid overload, which can lead to problems such as pulmonary edema. In severe cases, blood transfusions and intensive care may be necessary.

Dengue fever is a substantial public health challenge in many areas of the world, posing a hazard to millions of people living in tropical and subtropical countries. Understanding the complicated structure of the disease, including the four unique serotypes, transmission dynamics, and clinical symptoms, is critical for successful prevention, diagnosis, and management. Reducing the burden of dengue fever needs coordinated efforts in vector management, public education, early diagnosis, and fast treatment to lessen the impact of this potentially lethal disease.

Chapter 2

How Dengue Fever Spreads

Dengue fever is largely disseminated through the bite of infected female Aedes mosquitoes, notably Aedes aegypti and Aedes albopictus. These mosquitoes are particularly efficient vectors for the dengue virus, leading to the extensive transmission of the disease in tropical and subtropical countries. The transmission cycle of dengue involves both human hosts and mosquito vectors, with the virus being transferred back and forth between the two.

When an Aedes mosquito bites an individual infected with dengue, the mosquito ingests the virus along with the blood meal. The virus subsequently reaches the mosquito's midgut, where it begins to multiply. Over many days, the virus travels to the mosquito's salivary glands. Once the virus has reached the salivary glands, the mosquito becomes capable of transferring the infection to another human through its saliva during subsequent bites.

Mosquito Vectors and Transmission Dynamics

The principal vector of dengue fever is the Aedes aegypti mosquito, a species well suited to urban surroundings. Aedes aegypti mosquitoes can be identified by white markings on their legs and a marking in the form of a lyre on the upper surface of their thorax. These mosquitoes flourish close to human settlement, breeding in artificial containers that collect water, such as flower pots, abandoned tires, and water storage containers. Their life cycle, feeding habits, and behavior make them particularly successful at spreading dengue virus.

Breeding and Lifecycle: Aedes aegypti mosquitoes lay their eggs in clean, standing water. The eggs can tolerate desiccation for several months, allowing them to survive dry conditions. When water becomes available, the eggs hatch into larvae, which then develop into pupae and eventually emerge as adult mosquitoes. The full lifespan from egg to adult can be accomplished in as little as 8-10 days under optimal conditions. This fast lifetime, combined with the mosquito's penchant for mating in man-made containers, enables the growth of Aedes aegypti populations in urban environments.

Feeding Behavior: Aedes aegypti mosquitoes are daytime feeders, with peak biting activity happening in the early morning and late afternoon. They have a significant predilection for human blood, which boosts their efficacy as vectors of the dengue virus. Unlike many other mosquito species, Aedes aegypti mosquitoes are persistent biters and may feed numerous times in a single gonotrophic cycle (the period between blood meals during which eggs are formed and laid). This activity enhances the possibility of virus transmission, as an infected mosquito can bite numerous humans and disseminate the virus.

Resting and Movement: Aedes aegypti mosquitoes tend to rest indoors, frequently in dark, cool locations such as closets, beneath furniture, and behind curtains. Their short flight range, often less than 200 meters from their breeding grounds, means that dengue infection is often highly localized. However, human migration can contribute to the spread of the virus across wider distances, as infected persons might transport the virus to new places where they may be bitten by local mosquito populations.

Aedes albopictus: Although Aedes aegypti is the principal vector of the dengue virus, Aedes albopictus, popularly known as the Asian tiger mosquito, can also transmit the virus. Aedes albopictus is less anthropophilic (preferring human blood) than Aedes aegypti and is more prone to spawn in natural containers such as tree holes and bamboo stumps. This mosquito species is highly versatile and can survive in both urban and rural habitats. Aedes albopictus is capable of transmitting dengue virus, particularly in places where Aedes aegypti is less abundant or absent.

Role of Human Behavior in Transmission

Human behavior greatly determines the transmission dynamics of dengue illness. Factors such as population density, urbanization, water storage methods, and individual preventative measures all contribute to the likelihood of dengue transmission.

Population Density and Urbanization: High population density in urban areas produces optimal circumstances for the multiplication of Aedes aegypti mosquitoes and the spread of the dengue virus. Crowded living situations mean that a single sick mosquito can bite many individuals, increasing the risk of virus spread. Additionally, urbanization typically leads to the production of numerous artificial breeding habitats for mosquitoes, such as building sites, discarded containers, and poorly managed water storage systems.

Water Storage Practices: In many dengue-endemic countries, insufficient water supply infrastructure leads to the common habit of storing water in containers. These containers, if not adequately covered or maintained, become perfect breeding places for Aedes mosquitoes. Community education on adequate water storage practices, such as covering containers and routinely cleaning them to avoid mosquito breeding, is vital for minimizing the risk of dengue transmission.

Waste Management: Poor waste management techniques, such as the buildup of abandoned containers and tires, provide additional breeding places for Aedes mosquitoes. Effective waste management and community cleanup efforts can greatly reduce the number of potential mosquito breeding sites and lessen the risk of dengue transmission.

Individual Protective Measures: Personal protective measures play a significant role in minimizing the risk of mosquito bites and dengue transmission. Employing mosquito repellents, wearing long-sleeved clothing, and employing mosquito nets, particularly during peak biting times, can help protect humans from mosquito bites. Installing screens on windows and doors can also stop mosquitoes from accessing residential spaces. Public health initiatives that educate communities about these protective measures are vital for strengthening individual and community-level protection against dengue.

Travel and Movement: Human travel and movement contribute to the transmission of the dengue virus by moving infected persons to new places where local mosquito populations can become infected. This can lead to the transfer of the virus into previously unaffected locations, resulting in new outbreaks. Travelers to dengue-endemic areas should take steps to avoid mosquito bites and seek medical attention if they develop symptoms of dengue fever.

Community Engagement and Education: Community engagement and education are key components of dengue prevention and control activities. Public health initiatives that promote awareness about the transmission of dengue, the necessity of eliminating mosquito breeding areas, and the use of personal protective measures can empower communities to take proactive efforts to lower the risk of dengue. Engaging community leaders and local organizations in vector control activities can also boost the effectiveness of these projects.

Climate Change: Climate change can influence the transmission of dengue by influencing the range and number of mosquito vectors. Rising temperatures, altered precipitation patterns, and increased frequency of extreme weather events can produce more favorable conditions for mosquito breeding and virus replication. Understanding the influence of climate change on dengue transmission is critical for establishing adaptive measures to manage the evolving danger.

Public Health Infrastructure: The strength of public health infrastructure, including monitoring systems, diagnostic capability, and healthcare services, plays a significant role in controlling dengue outbreaks. Effective surveillance systems can detect and respond to epidemics promptly, while comprehensive diagnostic and healthcare services guarantee that patients receive timely and appropriate care. Investing in public health infrastructure is vital for lowering the impact of dengue and protecting vulnerable people.

Where the Mosquito-Driven Disease is Confirmed, Spreading Fastest

Dengue fever, principally carried by Aedes aegypti and Aedes albopictus mosquitoes, spreads swiftly in tropical and subtropical regions. The geographic expansion and intensity of dengue transmission are influenced by various factors, including climate, urbanization, and socioeconomic situations.

Southeast Asia: This region bears the highest burden of dengue globally. Countries like Thailand, Indonesia, the Philippines, and Vietnam report regular and severe outbreaks. The high population density, fast urbanization, and tropical climate with year-round warm temperatures and copious rains produce excellent circumstances for mosquito breeding and virus transmission. The cyclical pattern of dengue outbreaks in this region is driven by the persistent presence of all four dengue virus serotypes, leading to severe cases and high fatality rates.

Latin America and the Caribbean: Dengue fever is widespread across Latin America and the Caribbean, with nations such as Brazil, Mexico, Colombia, and Venezuela experiencing substantial public health challenges. Brazil, in particular, has seen a huge increase in dengue infections over the past decades, with repeated outbreaks affecting millions of people. The urbanization trend, combined with poor infrastructure and public health systems, exacerbates the transmission. Climate factors in these places also support mosquito proliferation, with seasonal rains generating numerous nesting grounds.

South Asia: India, Bangladesh, Pakistan, and Sri Lanka are among the South Asian countries that face significant dengue transmission rates. In India, dengue is a serious public health concern, with large-scale outbreaks occurring in both urban and rural areas. The monsoon season, with heavy rainfall and consequent waterlogging, provides abundant hatching grounds for Aedes mosquitoes. Inadequate water management and sanitation practices further enhance the development of dengue.

Western Pacific: The Western Pacific region, comprising nations such as Malaysia, Singapore, Australia, and the Pacific Islands, shows substantial dengue activity. Singapore, despite its modern healthcare infrastructure, has regular dengue epidemics due to its dense metropolitan population and suitable meteorological conditions. In Australia, dengue is limited to the northern regions, mainly Queensland, where the climate is appropriate for Aedes mosquito survival and reproduction.

Africa: Dengue is increasingly acknowledged as a public health problem in Africa. Countries like as Kenya, Tanzania, and Senegal have experienced outbreaks in recent years. The poor surveillance and diagnostic capabilities in many African nations mean that the true incidence of dengue is likely underestimated. However, increased urbanization, climate change, and worldwide travel are predicted to contribute to a surge in dengue transmission in the continent.

How Dengue Can Affect Your Brain and Nervous System

While dengue fever is mostly recognized for causing a febrile disease with symptoms such as high fever, severe headache, joint and muscular pain, and rash, it can also lead to severe brain consequences. These issues, although less prevalent, can have serious and long-lasting impacts on the brain and neurological system.

Dengue Encephalitis: Dengue encephalitis is a rare but serious consequence characterized by inflammation of the brain. Patients with dengue encephalitis may present with symptoms such as altered mental status, convulsions, severe headache, and localized neurological abnormalities. The pathophysiology of dengue encephalitis is not entirely understood; however, it is considered to result from direct viral invasion of the brain or an excessive immunological response to the infection. Diagnosis is typically based on clinical presentation, neuroimaging abnormalities, and laboratory testing to determine the presence of the dengue virus in cerebrospinal fluid (CSF). Management involves supportive care, seizure control, and methods to lower intracranial pressure.

Dengue Meningitis: Dengue meningitis involves inflammation of the meninges, the protective membranes surrounding the brain and spinal cord. Symptoms include severe headache, neck stiffness, photophobia (sensitivity to light), and disturbed mental status. The diagnosis is confirmed with lumbar puncture, which confirms a higher white blood cell count and the presence of the dengue virus in the CSF. Treatment is supportive and focused on treating symptoms and preventing complications.

Dengue Myelitis: Dengue myelitis, or inflammation of the spinal cord, can lead to symptoms such as weakness, paralysis, and sensory abnormalities. Patients may have acute flaccid paralysis, which can resemble poliomyelitis. The exact mechanism is unclear, but immune-mediated activities are considered to participate. Neuroimaging and CSF studies are critical for diagnosis, and management involves supportive care and physical therapy.

Guillain-Barré Syndrome (GBS): GBS is an autoimmune illness that can be induced by infections, including dengue. It is characterized by rapid-onset muscle weakness and paralysis that commonly begins in the legs and ascends to the upper body. The disorder occurs from the immune system attacking the peripheral nerves. Diagnosis is based on clinical presentation, nerve conduction testing, and CSF investigation indicative of high protein levels. Treatment includes intravenous immunoglobulin (IVIG) or plasmapheresis, and supportive treatment with strict monitoring for respiratory problems.

Dengue-Associated Acute Disseminated Encephalomyelitis (ADEM): ADEM is an inflammatory demyelinating disorder affecting the brain and spinal cord, commonly arising following viral infections like dengue. Symptoms include abrupt development of fever, headache, convulsions, and neurological impairments. MRI often indicates numerous inflammatory lesions in the brain and spinal cord. Treatment involves corticosteroids to reduce inflammation and supportive care to control symptoms.

Peripheral Neuropathy: Some dengue patients may develop peripheral neuropathy, characterized by numbness, tingling, and pain in the extremities. This disease can occur from direct viral injury to peripheral neurons or immune-mediated processes. Management focuses on symptom alleviation and physical rehabilitation.

Increased Risk of Dengue Virus in the United States

The risk of dengue virus infection in the United States has been growing due to various variables, including climate change, international travel, and the prevalence of Aedes mosquito populations. While dengue is not endemic to most parts of the United States, rare outbreaks and locally transmitted cases have been documented, notably in the southern states and territories such as Puerto Rico, the US Virgin Islands, and the Florida Keys.

Climate Change: Climate change has a substantial impact on the distribution and abundance of Aedes mosquitoes. Rising temperatures, more rainfall, and changes in weather patterns produce optimal conditions for mosquito breeding and survival. Warmer temperatures can curtail the mosquito development cycle and increase the number of mosquito bites, hence raising the possibility of dengue virus transmission. Regions of the United States with moderate winters and hot, humid summers are particularly vulnerable to the spread of dengue.

International Travel: The United States has a significant rate of international travel, with millions of people arriving from dengue-endemic locations each year. Infected travelers can spread the virus into local mosquito populations, leading to autochthonous (locally acquired) infections. Airports and big urban centers with high populations of international travelers are at increased risk for the introduction of dengue.

Presence of Aedes Mosquitoes: Aedes aegypti and Aedes albopictus mosquitoes are found in many parts of the United States, particularly in the southern states. These mosquitoes flourish in urban surroundings and are capable of transmitting the dengue virus if they bite an infected host. The presence of these vectors raises the possibility for local dengue transmission, particularly during the warmer months when mosquito activity is maximum.

Urbanization and Population Density: Urbanization and high population density in particular locations of the United States can facilitate the spread of dengue. Densely populated metropolitan environments provide various breeding habitats for Aedes mosquitoes, such as water-filled containers, abandoned tires, and poorly maintained water storage systems. Public health activities to reduce mosquito breeding areas and enhance waste management are vital for minimizing the risk of dengue transmission.

Public Health Preparedness: Public health preparedness and response play a crucial role in reducing dengue epidemics in the United States. Surveillance systems that monitor mosquito populations and detect dengue cases are critical for early detection and response to outbreaks. Public health programs that educate communities about mosquito control techniques and personal protective practices can also help minimize the risk of dengue transmission.

Limited Outbreaks: The United States has experienced limited outbreaks of dengue in recent years. For example, Florida has reported many outbreaks, with locally transmitted cases occurring in Miami-Dade County and the Florida Keys. Texas has also known rare occurrences of locally transmitted dengue. These outbreaks underline the need for ongoing monitoring and public health efforts to prevent and manage dengue transmission.

Healthcare System and Diagnostic Capacity: The United States has a solid healthcare system and diagnostic capacity, which facilitates timely diagnosis and management of dengue cases. Rapid diagnostic methods, molecular assays, and serological testing are available to detect the dengue virus and identify individual serotypes. Prompt diagnosis and supportive care are critical for managing dengue patients and preventing serious sequelae.

Public Awareness and Education: Raising public awareness of dengue prevention and control is vital for minimizing the risk of infection. Public health initiatives that provide information on how to reduce mosquito breeding areas, use insect repellents, and guard against mosquito bites can empower individuals and communities to take proactive measures. Engaging community leaders and local groups in these activities can boost the effectiveness of public health programs.

The increased risk of dengue virus infection in the United States is impacted by factors such as climate change, foreign travel, the presence of Aedes mosquitoes, urbanization, and public health preparedness. Addressing these elements through extensive surveillance, vector control, public awareness, and healthcare infrastructure is critical for preventing and controlling dengue transmission.

Chapter 3

Signs and Symptoms

Dengue fever is a mosquito-borne epidemiologic infection that can cause a range of symptoms, from mild to severe. The clinical presentation of dengue fever can vary substantially, making it necessary to recognize the signs and symptoms for a correct diagnosis and appropriate treatment.

Common Symptoms of Dengue Fever

The incubation time for dengue fever normally ranges from 4 to 10 days after the bite of an infected mosquito. The disease can manifest on a spectrum, from mild febrile sickness to severe and possibly life-threatening forms such as dengue hemorrhagic fever (DHF) and dengue shock syndrome (DSS). The common signs of dengue fever include:

Fever: The characteristic of dengue fever is a sudden onset of high fever, classically reaching up to 104°F (40°C). This fever is frequently biphasic or saddleback in character, where the fever drops after a few days and then returns.

Severe Headache: A severe and frequently excruciating headache, generally centered behind the eyes (retro-orbital pain), is a common symptom. This headache is generally accompanied by pain in the eyes.

Joint and Muscle Pain: Dengue fever is generally referred to as "breakbone fever" because of the terrible muscle and joint pains it causes. This pain can be so acute that it feels like the bones are cracking.

Rash: A rash commonly appears two to five days following the onset of fever. The rash might vary in appearance; however, it is frequently described as a maculopapular or petechial rash. It often starts on the trunk and extends to the limbs and face.

Nausea and Vomiting: Many patients report gastrointestinal symptoms such as nausea, vomiting, and loss of appetite. These symptoms can contribute to dehydration, especially in youngsters.

Weariness and Weakness: Severe weariness and generalized weakness are frequent during the acute phase of the illness and can remain for several weeks during recovery.

Pain Behind the Eyes: Pain behind the eyes is a specific and common symptom of dengue fever, contributing to the total pain experienced by patients.

Swollen Glands: Some individuals may develop lymphadenopathy, or swollen glands, as a response to the viral infection.

Differences in Symptoms Among Age Groups and Regions

The clinical signs of dengue fever can vary based on the age of the patient and the geographical region. Understanding these variations is critical for accurate diagnosis and management.

Newborns and Young Children: In newborns and young children, dengue fever generally manifests with nonspecific symptoms that can resemble other common viral diseases. These symptoms include fever, rash, and upper respiratory problems. Young children may also develop irritability and unwillingness to feed. Due to their incapacity to verbalize particular symptoms, the diagnosis of dengue in this age range might be hard. Additionally, infants may be at higher risk for severe types of dengue due to their developing immune systems.

Older Children and Teenagers: Older children and teenagers tend to develop more characteristic symptoms of dengue fever, such as high fever, severe headache, joint and muscular discomfort, and rash. However, they may also be more prone to serious problems, including DHF and DSS. The intensity of symptoms can be modified by prior exposure to various dengue virus serotypes, as secondary infections are associated with a higher risk of severe disease.

Adults: Adults often present with the entire spectrum of dengue symptoms, including high fever, headache, retro-orbital pain, joint and muscle pain, rash, and gastrointestinal symptoms. In adults, severe dengue can lead to major morbidity, with consequences such as plasma leakage, hemorrhage, and organ damage. Comorbidities and underlying health issues can aggravate the severity of the disease in adulthood.

Regional Variations: The clinical presentation of dengue can also vary by region due to changes in dengue virus serotypes, vector populations, and environmental factors. For instance, in places where many serotypes circulate, the risk of severe dengue increases due to the phenomenon of antibody-dependent enhancement (ADE). ADE occurs when a person previously infected with one serotype is infected with a different serotype, leading to a more severe immunological response. Additionally, genetic and immunological factors can influence how individuals from different regions respond to dengue illness.

Risk Factors for Severe Cases

Several risk factors are connected with the development of severe dengue, including DHF and DSS. Identifying these risk factors is critical for predicting the course of the disease and providing appropriate medical care.

Previous Dengue Infection: One of the most significant risk factors for severe dengue is a previous infection with a different serotype of the dengue virus. Secondary infections are more likely to result in severe disease due to ADE, where non-neutralizing antibodies from the initial infection promote the uptake of the virus into immune cells, resulting in an exaggerated immunological response.

Age: Age is a major factor in dengue severity. Infants and young children are at higher risk for severe dengue due to their undeveloped immune systems. Additionally, the aged population may have more severe disease due to age-related changes in immunity and the prevalence of comorbidities.

Comorbidities: Individuals with underlying medical problems such as diabetes, hypertension, heart disease, and chronic renal disease are at increased risk for severe dengue. These problems can exacerbate the course of the disease and make management more complicated.

Pregnancy: Pregnant women are at higher risk for severe dengue and bad pregnancy outcomes. Dengue infection during pregnancy can lead to issues such as preterm birth, low birth weight, and potentially mother and fetal death. Close monitoring and supportive care are needed for pregnant women with dengue.

Genetic Factors: Genetic predisposition can influence the severity of dengue. Certain genetic variations in immune response genes have been related to greater vulnerability to severe dengue. Understanding these genetic characteristics can help identify those at higher risk and advise individualized medical care.

Nutritional Status: Malnutrition, particularly in children, might weaken the immune response and increase vulnerability to severe dengue. Conversely, obesity has also been found to be a risk factor for severe dengue, probably due to impaired immune function and the presence of chronic inflammation.

Gender: Some research suggests that females may be at increased risk for severe dengue compared to males. The reasons for this discrepancy are not understood but may involve hormonal and immunological issues.

Viral Factors: The virulence of the dengue virus strain can also influence disease severity. Certain strains are more likely to produce severe disease, and the genetic variety of the virus adds to variances in clinical presentation.

Socioeconomic Factors: Socioeconomic factors such as access to healthcare, quality of housing, and public health infrastructure have a key effect on dengue outcomes. Poor living conditions, inadequate water management, and restricted access to medical treatment might raise the risk of severe dengue.

Timing of Medical Care: Early recognition and appropriate medical care are critical for preventing serious dengue sequelae. Delays in obtaining medical attention or misdiagnosis can lead to worse results.

Public awareness initiatives and training for healthcare personnel are vital for improving early diagnosis and management.

Environmental Factors: Environmental circumstances, particularly climate and weather patterns, influence the breeding and activity of Aedes mosquitoes. Regions with high humidity and frequent rainfall are more conducive to mosquito development, increasing the likelihood of dengue transmission and severe epidemics.

Immune Response: The host immune response to dengue infection plays a vital role in disease severity. An excessive or dysregulated immune response can lead to problems such as plasma leakage, hemorrhage, and organ failure. Understanding the immunological processes involved in dengue pathogenesis is critical for developing targeted treatments.

Diagnostic Methods: Antibody Detection, PCR, and Viral Isolation

Accurate and fast diagnosis of dengue fever is critical for optimal clinical care and the prevention of serious sequelae. Several diagnostic procedures are available to detect dengue virus infection, each with its advantages and limits. The three primary diagnostic techniques are antibody detection, polymerase chain reaction (PCR), and viral isolation.

Antibody Detection: Serological assays are routinely used to detect antibodies generated in response to dengue virus infection. There are two main types of antibodies detected: immunoglobulin M (IgM) and Immunoglobulin G (IgG).

IgM Antibodies: IgM antibodies are the first antibodies produced by the immune system in response to a dengue infection. They usually occur within 3 to 5 days following the onset of symptoms and can be detected for several weeks. IgM detection is effective for diagnosing recent infections. The enzyme-linked immunosorbent test (ELISA) is the most extensively used method for detecting IgM antibodies. Rapid diagnostic tests (RDTs) are also available for point-of-care testing, yielding results within 15 to 30 minutes. However, IgM tests can cross-react with other flaviviruses, such as Zika and West Nile, potentially leading to false-positive results.

IgG Antibodies: IgG antibodies emerge later in the course of the infection, usually around the second week of illness, and persist for life. The detection of IgG antibodies is useful for identifying prior dengue infections and for seroepidemiological studies. A large increase in IgG titers between acute and convalescent tests can indicate a recent infection. The plaque reduction neutralization test (PRNT) is the gold typical for quantifying dengue-specific neutralizing antibodies; however, it is more labor-intensive and time-consuming compared to ELISA.

Polymerase Chain Reaction (PCR): PCR is a molecular technique used to detect viral RNA in blood or other clinical specimens. Reverse transcription PCR (RT-PCR) is extensively used for dengue diagnosis. PCR can detect the virus during the acute phase of the illness, often during the first 5 to 7 days after symptoms start. This approach is highly sensitive and specific, allowing for the determination of the dengue virus serotype. Real-time PCR (qPCR) gives quantitative results and faster processing times. PCR is very effective in identifying dengue from other febrile diseases with similar clinical manifestations. However, the demand for specialized laboratory equipment and technical skills limits its availability in resource-constrained situations.

Viral Isolation: Viral isolation entails growing the dengue virus from clinical samples, such as blood or serum, in cell lines. This method gives definitive evidence of dengue infection and enables additional study on viral properties and behavior. Viral isolation is primarily performed in reference laboratories and is employed for research purposes rather than routine diagnosis due to its complexity and longer turnaround time. Cell culture techniques, such as C6/36 mosquito cell lines or Vero cells, are extensively employed for dengue virus isolation. Once isolated, the virus can be identified by immunofluorescence or PCR.

Differential Diagnosis to Rule Out Other Febrile Illnesses

Dengue fever has symptoms similar to those of many other febrile infections, making differential diagnosis necessary to ensure correct diagnosis and proper treatment. Clinicians must examine a spectrum of different diseases that present with similar clinical characteristics, especially in regions where several infectious diseases are endemic.

Malaria: Malaria and dengue fever can both look as high fever, headache, and muscle pain. However, malaria often causes recurring fever spikes (every 48 to 72 hours) along with chills and sweating, which are less common in dengue. Thick and thin blood smears for microscopic examination or fast diagnostic tests for malaria antigens are utilized to differentiate malaria from dengue.

Zika Virus: Zika virus infection, like dengue, is transmitted by Aedes mosquitoes and shares symptoms such as fever, rash, and joint discomfort. However, Zika typically causes conjunctivitis and is associated with serious congenital defects if infection occurs during pregnancy. PCR and serological assays are used to distinguish Zika from dengue, recognizing the potential for cross-reactivity.

Chikungunya: Chikungunya virus infection also manifests with high fever and severe joint pain, similar to dengue. However, joint pain in chikungunya tends to be stronger and more protracted, commonly affecting the tiny joints of the hands and feet. PCR and serological tests can identify Chikungunya from dengue.

Leptospirosis: Leptospirosis, a bacterial infection acquired through contact with contaminated water or soil, can mirror dengue symptoms, including fever, headache, and muscle discomfort. Leptospirosis might also induce jaundice, renal failure, and bleeding. Serological assays (ELISA or microscopic agglutination test) and PCR are used to detect leptospirosis.

Typhoid Fever: Typhoid fever, caused by Salmonella Typhi, presents with persistent fever, abdominal pain, and gastrointestinal symptoms, which can overlap with dengue. Blood cultures or serological tests (widal tests) help diagnose typhoid fever.

Influenza: Influenza and dengue share symptoms such as fever, headache, and muscle pain. Influenza generally includes respiratory symptoms including cough and sore throat, which are less common in dengue. Quick antigen tests and PCR can confirm influenza.

Rickettsial Infections: Rickettsial diseases, including scrub typhus and spotted fever, can present with fever, headache, rash, and myalgia, similar to dengue. Specific serological testing, or PCR, is necessary for diagnosis.

Yellow Fever: Yellow fever, another flavivirus spread by Aedes mosquitoes, can cause fever, headache, and jaundice. Yellow fever vaccination status and particular serological testing (ELISA or PCR) help identify it as dengue.

Hepatitis: Viral hepatitis (A, B, C, E) can induce fever, tiredness, and jaundice, resembling severe dengue. Liver function testing and serological markers for hepatitis viruses subsidize to the diagnosis.

COVID-19: COVID-19, caused by the SARS-CoV-2 virus, shares some overlapping symptoms with dengue, such as fever, headache, and myalgia. COVID-19 often includes respiratory symptoms like coughing and shortness of breath. PCR tests for SARS-CoV-2 and serological tests for COVID-19 antibodies are used for diagnosis.

Diagnostic Approach: When a patient presents with symptoms suggestive of dengue, clinicians follow a systematic approach to diagnosis:

Clinical Assessment: Evaluate the patient's symptoms, onset and duration of illness, and any recent travel to dengue-endemic areas.

Epidemiological Context: Consider local dengue transmission patterns and outbreak reports.

Laboratory Testing: Utilize appropriate laboratory tests based on the phase of the illness:

Early Phase (0–5 days): NS1 antigen detection or PCR to detect viral RNA.

Later Phase (5+ days): Serological tests for IgM and IgG antibodies.

Differential Diagnosis: Rule out other febrile illnesses with overlapping symptoms using specific laboratory tests and clinical criteria.

Detailed Discussion on Specific Tests

NS1 Antigen Test: The NS1 antigen test is particularly valuable during the early phase of dengue infection. It can detect the presence of the dengue virus as early as the first day of symptoms and up to day 9. This test's rapid results aid in early diagnosis and timely patient management, reducing the risk of severe complications. While NS1 antigen tests are highly specific, they may have varying sensitivity depending on the serotype and patient population. Combining NS1 antigen testing with antibody detection enhances diagnostic accuracy.

IgM/IgG Antibody Tests: Serological tests for IgM and IgG antibodies provide essential information on the patient's immune response to dengue infection. IgM antibodies specify recent infection, while IgG antibodies suggest past exposure or secondary infection. In primary dengue infections, IgM antibodies typically appear by day 5 and peak around day 14. IgG antibodies appear advanced and persist for life. In secondary infections, IgG antibodies rise rapidly and to higher levels, while IgM response may be weaker or absent. Serological tests are particularly useful in later stages of illness when viral components are no longer detectable.

PCR for Dengue RNA: PCR is the gold standard for early diagnosis of dengue infection. It can detect viral RNA in blood or other clinical specimens within the first few days of illness. PCR allows for the identification of dengue virus serotypes, which is valuable for epidemiological surveillance and understanding disease dynamics. Real-time PCR (qPCR) offers quantitative results and faster processing times, enhancing its utility in clinical and public health settings. PCR's high sensitivity and specificity make it an indispensable tool for early and accurate dengue diagnosis.

Differential Diagnosis in Practice: Given the overlap in clinical features between dengue and other febrile illnesses, differential diagnosis is a critical component of patient evaluation. Clinicians must consider various factors, including:

Travel History: Recent travel to dengue-endemic areas increases the likelihood of dengue infection.

Seasonal Patterns: Dengue outbreaks often follow seasonal patterns, with higher transmission during the rainy season when mosquito populations increase.

Clinical Features: Specific symptoms, such as retro-orbital pain, severe myalgia, and petechial rash, may suggest dengue. Nevertheless, overlapping symptoms with other diseases necessitate laboratory confirmation.

Laboratory Results: Combining clinical evaluation with laboratory tests, such as NS1 antigen, IgM/IgG antibodies, and PCR, provides a comprehensive diagnostic approach. Negative results for one test should prompt consideration of other diagnostic methods or repeat testing if clinical suspicion remains high.

An accurate diagnosis of dengue fever relies on a combination of clinical assessment and laboratory testing. The use of NS1 antigen detection, PCR for viral RNA, and serological tests for IgM and IgG antibodies enables timely and accurate diagnosis, distinguishing dengue from other febrile illnesses. A systematic diagnostic approach ensures appropriate patient management, reduces the risk of severe complications, and supports effective public health interventions.

Warning Signs and Complications

Recognizing the warning signals of severe dengue and its consequences is vital for reducing morbidity and mortality. Dengue fever can escalate to severe forms, such as dengue hemorrhagic fever (DHF) and dengue shock syndrome (DSS), which require prompt medical intervention.

Warning Signs: During the crucial period, usually occurring around the time of defervescence (when the fever declines), patients may exhibit warning signs indicating a risk of severe dengue. These signs include:

Severe stomach pain: Intense and chronic stomach pain can suggest internal hemorrhage or organ involvement.

Persistent Vomiting: Continuous vomiting leads to dehydration and might be a sign of gastrointestinal bleeding or severe sickness.

Mucosal Bleeding: Bleeding from the gums, nose, or other mucosal surfaces indicates coagulopathy or severe dengue.

Lethargy or Restlessness: Extreme weariness or irritability can signify oncoming shock or severe sickness.

Hepatomegaly: Enlargement of the liver, typically combined with soreness, might signify a severe illness.

Fluid Accumulation: Clinical signs of fluid accumulation, such as pleural effusion (fluid in the chest cavity) or ascites (fluid in the belly), suggest plasma leakage and severe dengue.

Laboratory Findings: Laboratory tests revealing a rapid reduction in platelet count (thrombocytopenia), an increase in hematocrit (hemoconcentration), or abnormal liver function tests suggest severe dengue.

Consequences: Severe dengue can lead to various life-threatening consequences that require rapid medical intervention:

Dengue Hemorrhagic Fever (DHF): DHF is characterized by plasma leakage, hemorrhage, and thrombocytopenia. The plasma leakage might lead to hypovolemia (lower blood volume) and shock if not handled promptly. DHF is divided into four grades (I-IV) according to severity, with grades III and IV implying DSS. Bleeding signs might range from moderate (petechiae and bruises) to severe (gastrointestinal bleeding and cerebral hemorrhage).

Dengue Shock Syndrome (DSS): DSS is the most severe type of dengue, resulting from substantial plasma leakage leading to shock. Shock appears with a quick, weak pulse; hypotension (low blood pressure); cold, clammy skin; and restlessness. Immediate fluid resuscitation and supportive care are necessary to manage shock and prevent organ failure.

Organ Involvement: Severe dengue can include numerous organs, leading to consequences such as:

Liver: Severe liver involvement might result in hepatitis, liver failure, and coagulopathy.

Kidneys: Acute kidney damage (AKI) can develop owing to dehydration, shock, or direct viral impacts.

Heart: Myocarditis (inflammation of the heart muscle) and heart failure can produce.

Lungs: Pulmonary edema (fluid accumulation in the lungs) and acute respiratory distress syndrome (ARDS) can occur owing to plasma leakage.

Brain: Neurological problems, such as encephalopathy, seizures, and coma, can arise with severe dengue.

Management of Severe Dengue: The management of severe dengue entails supportive care and surveillance to avoid and treat complications. Key aspects of management include:

Fluid Management: Intravenous (IV) fluid therapy is needed to maintain proper blood volume and prevent shock. The type and volume of fluid provided are carefully monitored depending on clinical assessment and test findings. Balanced crystalloids are normally utilized, while colloids may be explored in severe shock.

Hemodynamic Monitoring: Continuous monitoring of vital signs, urine output, and hematocrit levels is necessary to assess the patient's response to fluid therapy and detect early signs of shock.

Blood Transfusions: In cases of severe bleeding or profound thrombocytopenia, blood transfusions, including platelet concentrates, may be indicated.

Oxygen Therapy: Supplemental oxygen is supplied to individuals with respiratory distress or hypoxemia (low blood oxygen levels).

Management of Coagulopathy: Coagulation disorders are handled with suitable blood products and drugs as needed.

Monitoring for problems: Regular assessment for signs of organ involvement and problems is crucial to providing prompt interventions.

The diagnosis and therapy of dengue fever involve a multidimensional approach, including reliable diagnostic procedures, differential diagnosis to rule out other febrile infections, and vigilant monitoring for warning signs and sequelae. Early detection and effective medical care are crucial to improving outcomes and minimizing the burden of this potentially life-threatening disease.

Chapter 4

Diagnosis and Testing

Accurate diagnosis of dengue fever is crucial for effective patient management and public health interventions. The complexity of dengue's clinical presentation, which often overlaps with other febrile illnesses, necessitates the use of various diagnostic methods and laboratory tests. Understanding the strengths and limitations of these methods ensures appropriate and timely diagnosis, enabling better clinical outcomes and disease control.

Methods for Diagnosing Dengue Fever

Diagnosing dengue fever involves a combination of clinical evaluation, patient history, and laboratory tests. Clinicians must consider the epidemiological context, including recent travel to dengue-endemic areas, and the presence of specific signs and symptoms such as high fever, severe headache, retro-orbital pain, myalgia, arthralgia, rash, and hemorrhagic manifestations. The following are the primary methods used for diagnosing dengue fever:

Clinical Diagnosis: In endemic areas, the clinical diagnosis of dengue fever is often based on the patient's symptoms and signs, combined with a history of exposure to mosquito bites. The World Health Organization (WHO) has provided guiding principle to assist clinicians in recognizing dengue, including the identification of warning signs for severe dengue. However, clinical diagnosis alone can be challenging due to the nonspecific nature of early symptoms and their similarity to other febrile illnesses.

Laboratory Diagnosis: Laboratory tests play a critical role in confirming dengue virus infection and distinguishing it from other diseases. The primary laboratory methods include:

Detection of Dengue Virus or its Components: This involves detecting viral components such as the NS1 antigen or viral RNA during the acute phase of the infection.

Serological Tests: These tests detect the patient's immune response to the dengue virus by identifying specific antibodies (IgM and IgG).

Laboratory Tests (NS1 Antigen, IgM/IgG Antibodies)

NS1 Antigen Detection: The nonstructural protein 1 (NS1) antigen is a component of the dengue virus that can be detected in the blood during the early stages of infection. NS1 antigen detection tests, including ELISA (enzyme-linked immunosorbent assay) and rapid diagnostic tests (RDTs), are highly sensitive and specific. These tests are particularly useful in the first few days after the onset of symptoms, before the appearance of detectable antibodies.

ELISA for NS1: The ELISA test for NS1 antigen is commonly used in laboratory settings. It can provide results within a few hours and is capable of detecting NS1 antigen in both primary and secondary dengue infections. The high specificity of the ELISA test helps distinguish dengue from other febrile illnesses.

Rapid Diagnostic Tests (RDTs) for NS1: RDTs offer a convenient and quick method for detecting the NS1 antigen, providing results within 15–30 minutes. These tests are especially useful in resource-limited settings and for point-of-care testing. While RDTs are generally less sensitive than ELISA, they are valuable for early diagnosis and prompt patient management.

IgM and IgG Antibody Detection: Serological tests detect dengue-specific antibodies produced by the immune system in response to infection. IgM antibodies are the first to appear, followed by IgG antibodies.

IgM Antibodies: IgM antibodies typically appear 3-5 days after the onset of symptoms and indicate a recent infection. The presence of IgM antibodies is a strong indicator of acute dengue infection. IgM antibodies can be detected using ELISA or immunochromatographic assays (rapid tests). These tests are widely available and easy to perform.

IgG Antibodies: IgG antibodies appear later, usually around the second week of illness, and remain detectable for life. IgG detection is useful for identifying past infections and assessing immunity. In cases of secondary dengue infection, IgG antibodies rise rapidly and to higher levels compared to primary infections. The plaque reduction neutralization test (PRNT) is considered the gold standard for measuring dengue-specific neutralizing antibodies, though it is more labor-intensive and time-consuming than other serological tests.

Chapter 5

Treatment and Management

Dengue fever is a viral virus that is transmitted by mosquitoes and offers considerable problems to public health, particularly in tropical and subtropical locations all over the world. It is necessary to have treatment and management options that are effective to reduce the impact that the disease has on populations that are impacted. If you want to improve patient outcomes and prevent serious consequences, supportive care and careful management of symptoms are essential. Although there is no particular antiviral treatment for dengue fever, supportive care and careful management of symptoms are essential.

Options for Treatment Currently

Available for Dengue Fever

Due to the absence of a specific antiviral drug that specifically targets the dengue virus, the primary focus of treatment for dengue fever is on providing supportive care. Among the crucial therapy choices are:

Fluid Management: Maintaining an appropriate level of hydration is essential for treating dengue fever. Patients suffering from dengue fever that is mild to moderate should be advised to consume a large number of fluids to avoid becoming dehydrated. Oral rehydration solutions, often known as ORS, are particularly useful for preventing dehydration and preserving the electrolyte balance of the body. When the patient's condition is severe, it may be required to administer fluids through an intravenous (IV) line to ensure that they are adequately hydrated and to stabilize their state.

Fever and Pain Management: Antipyretics and analgesics are routinely used to treat fever and alleviate pain. Paracetamol (acetaminophen) is the chosen drug for fever control and pain relief in dengue patients. Non-steroidal anti-inflammatory medicines (NSAIDs), such as ibuprofen and aspirin, should be avoided as they can increase the risk of bleeding and aggravate the clinical course of dengue.

Rest and Monitoring: Patients diagnosed with dengue fever should be recommended to rest and avoid intense activities. Regular monitoring of vital signs, such as temperature, blood pressure, and pulse rate, is needed to detect early signs of worsening and avert serious problems.

Supportive Care and Symptom Management

Supportive care is the foundation stone of dengue fever treatment, focused on treating symptoms and preventing complications. The main components of supportive care include:

Hydration: Adequate fluid intake is necessary to prevent dehydration, which can worsen the severity of dengue fever. Patients should be urged to drink water, oral rehydration solutions, and clear fluids. In circumstances where oral intake is insufficient or the patient is unable to drink, IV fluids should be delivered under medical supervision.

Pain and Fever Relief: Paracetamol is advised for managing fever and alleviating pain. It is recommended to avoid NSAIDs and aspirin due to their potential to cause gastrointestinal bleeding and other hemorrhagic problems. Paracetamol can be taken every 4–6 hours, with careful monitoring of the total daily dosage to minimize hepatotoxicity.

Monitoring and Rest: Patients should be observed for changes in symptoms and any signs of worsening. Regular measurement of vital signs, such as blood pressure, heart rate, and temperature, helps spot issues early. Rest is vital for recovery, and patients should be encouraged to minimize physical effort.

Diet & Nutrition: Maintaining a balanced diet is vital for general health and recuperation. Patients should have light, nutritious meals that are easy to digest. In cases of severe dengue, where gastrointestinal symptoms such as nausea and vomiting are present, IV fluids and nutrition may be required.

Guidelines for Managing Severe Cases (Dengue Hemorrhagic Fever and Dengue Shock Syndrome)

Severe dengue infections, including dengue hemorrhagic fever (DHF) and dengue shock syndrome (DSS), require specific therapy to address the increased risk of complications and fatality. The following guidelines define the strategy for handling severe cases:

Hospitalization and Intense Care: Patients with severe dengue should be hospitalized for close observation and intense care. Early identification and quick management are critical to preventing problems and enhancing outcomes.

Fluid Management: Fluid therapy is the foundation of treatment for severe dengue. The goal is to keep enough blood volume and prevent shock. Isotonic crystalloids, such as normal saline or Ringer's lactate, are often utilized. Fluid delivery should be closely controlled to avoid overhydration, which can lead to fluid overload and respiratory distress. The following stages are normally followed:

Initial Resuscitation: Rapid fluid boluses (10–20 ml/kg) are provided to stabilize the patient's condition and improve perfusion.

Maintenance Phase: Once the patient is stable, fluid delivery is regulated based on clinical factors and laboratory results, such as hematocrit and urine output. The rate of fluid administration is gradually lowered to avoid fluid excess.

Monitoring: Regular monitoring of vital signs, urine output, hematocrit, and other clinical markers is crucial to guide fluid management and detect problems early.

Blood Transfusion: In cases of major bleeding or severe thrombocytopenia (low platelet count), blood transfusions may be indicated. Platelet transfusions are indicated for individuals with active bleeding and very low platelet counts. Fresh frozen plasma or packed red blood cells may be delivered to control severe bleeding and preserve hemodynamic stability.

Monitoring for issues: Close monitoring is crucial to discovering issues early and intervening swiftly. Key complications to monitor include:

Bleeding: Gastrointestinal bleeding, epistaxis (nosebleeds), and bleeding gums are typical in severe dengue. Regular examination of bleeding tendencies and coagulation markers helps control bleeding issues efficiently.

Organ Involvement: Severe dengue can damage several organs, leading to consequences such as hepatitis, myocarditis, encephalopathy, and renal failure. Regular monitoring of liver and kidney function tests, heart indicators, and neurological examinations is required.

Shock: Dengue shock syndrome (DSS) is a life-threatening disorder characterized by extreme hypotension and poor perfusion. Early detection and intensive fluid resuscitation are crucial to preventing permanent shock and organ failure.

Monitoring for Complications

Monitoring for complications is an important feature of dengue management, particularly in severe infections. Regular examinations and appropriate therapies can prevent the advancement of the disease and enhance patient outcomes. The following are critical factors for monitoring complications:

Vital Signs: Continuous monitoring of vital signs, including blood pressure, heart rate, breathing rate, and temperature, helps detect early signs of deterioration. Hypotension, tachycardia, and fever spikes may suggest consequences such as shock, hemorrhage, or secondary infections.

Hematocrit: Monitoring hematocrit levels helps measure the patient's hydration state and detect hemoconcentration, which can suggest plasma leakage. Rising hematocrit levels may signify approaching shock and the need for additional fluid delivery.

Platelet Count: Regular monitoring of platelet counts is necessary to determine the risk of bleeding and advise on the need for platelet transfusions. Severe thrombocytopenia (platelet count < 20,000 cells/µL) increases the risk of spontaneous bleeding and requires strict surveillance.

Liver Function Tests: Elevated liver enzymes (ALT and AST) suggest hepatic involvement and can assist in assessing the severity of liver disease. Severe hepatitis may require further supportive measures and monitoring.

Renal Function Tests: Monitoring renal function (creatinine and blood urea nitrogen levels) is critical to detect acute kidney injury and guide fluid management. Renal failure may demand modifications in fluid treatment and other supportive measures.

Clinical Assessment: Regular clinical exams assist in discovering problems and guide treatment recommendations. Key parts of clinical assessment include:

Hydration state: Assessing the patient's hydration state by clinical indicators (e.g., skin turgor, mucous membranes, urine output) helps guide fluid therapy and prevent dehydration or fluid overload.

Bleeding Tendencies: Evaluating bleeding tendencies (e.g., petechiae, ecchymosis, mucosal bleeding) helps determine the likelihood of hemorrhagic consequences and indicates the need for blood transfusions.

Organ Involvement: Assessing symptoms of organ involvement (e.g., jaundice, altered mental status, chest pain) can help discover problems such as hepatitis, encephalopathy, and myocarditis. Early detection and intervention are critical to preventing organ failure.

Imaging investigations: In certain circumstances, imaging investigations such as ultrasound or chest X-ray may be indicated to assess problems such as pleural effusion, ascites, or pulmonary edema. These examinations provide crucial information to guide treatment decisions and evaluate the development of the disease.

Effective treatment and management of dengue fever require a comprehensive approach that includes supportive care, diligent monitoring, and prompt treatments. By adhering to established recommendations and protocols, healthcare providers can improve patient outcomes, lower the risk of severe sequelae, and mitigate the impact of dengue fever on impacted populations.

When to Seek Medical Attention

Recognizing when to seek medical assistance for dengue fever is critical for timely intervention and averting serious consequences. Dengue fever can range from mild to severe, and understanding the warning signals is critical for patients and caregivers.

Severe stomach pain or prolonged Vomiting: Severe and prolonged stomach pain, especially if it is accompanied by vomiting, can indicate dengue hemorrhagic fever (DHF) or dengue shock syndrome (DSS). These symptoms imply potential consequences, such as plasma leakage, which might lead to shock if not treated swiftly.

Bleeding: Any indicators of bleeding, such as nosebleeds, gum bleeding, or blood in vomit or stool, need rapid medical attention. Petechiae (small red or purple spots on the skin) and easy bruising are further concerning indicators that should not be overlooked.

Weariness and Restlessness: Severe weariness, restlessness, or irritability may suggest shock or other serious consequences. These symptoms can be minor but are vital markers of the body's stress and need for medical assessment.

Rapid Breathing: Increased respiratory rate or difficulty breathing might be a sign of fluid accumulation in the lungs (pulmonary edema) or other complications connected to severe dengue. Immediate medical intervention is important to handle these problems.

Decreased Urine Output: A considerable decline in urine output is a symptom of dehydration or renal dysfunction. Monitoring urine output is an efficient technique to measure hydration status and kidney function.

Avoiding Aspirin and NSAIDs Due to Bleeding Risk

Managing pain and fever in dengue patients involves the cautious selection of drugs to avoid complications. Aspirin and non-steroidal anti-inflammatory medicines (NSAIDs) such as ibuprofen and naproxen should be avoided due to their propensity to increase bleeding risk.

Why Aspirin and NSAIDs Are Risky: Aspirin and NSAIDs reduce platelet activity and can cause gastrointestinal discomfort, all of which increase the risk of bleeding in dengue patients. Given that dengue can cause thrombocytopenia (low platelet count), utilizing these drugs exacerbates the risk of bleeding.

Recommended Alternatives: Paracetamol (acetaminophen) is the ideal drug for controlling fever and pain in dengue patients. It does not influence platelet function and has a lesser risk of producing gastrointestinal bleeding. The dosage should be closely controlled to avoid hepatotoxicity, especially in youngsters.

Fluid Management and Pain Relief

Fluid management and pain reduction are key parts of dengue fever treatment, focusing on preserving hydration and providing comfort to the patient.

Fluid Management: Proper hydration is crucial for dengue patients to prevent dehydration and control symptoms. Patients should be encouraged to drink plenty of fluids, such as water, oral rehydration treatments, and clear soups. In severe situations, intravenous (IV) fluids may be indicated.

Oral Rehydration: For patients with mild to moderate symptoms, oral rehydration solutions (ORS) are beneficial in preserving electrolyte balance and preventing dehydration. These solutions include the correct balance of salts and carbohydrates to enhance absorption in the gut.

Fluids: In cases of severe dehydration or when oral intake is insufficient, IV fluid delivery is essential. Isotonic crystalloids, such as normal saline or Ringer's lactate, are often utilized. Fluid delivery should be carefully controlled to avoid fluid excess, which can lead to problems such as pulmonary edema.

Pain Relief: Managing pain successfully increases patient comfort and can promote recovery. Paracetamol is the medicine of choice for alleviating pain and decreasing temperature. The prescribed dosage should be adhered to, with a maximum of 4 grams per day for adults and reduced dosages for children based on weight.

Long-Term Effects and Post-Dengue Syndrome

While most dengue patients recover totally within a few weeks, others may endure long-term complications, known as post-dengue syndrome. This disorder might include a spectrum of symptoms that continue long after the acute phase of the sickness has resolved.

Weariness and Weakness: Many patients describe chronic weariness and overall weakness, which can linger for weeks or even months. This post-viral weariness is comparable to what is seen in other viral illnesses and can influence everyday activities and quality of life.

Joint and Muscle Pain: Some patients endure persistent joint and muscle pain, a disease known as arthralgia. This pain can be debilitating and may require continuing pain management techniques, such as physical therapy or drugs.

Depression and Anxiety: The physical impact of dengue, along with the stress of severe sickness, can rise to psychological repercussions such as depression and anxiety. Mental health help and therapy may be important for certain patients to cope with these issues.

Neurological Effects: Although rare, some people may have neurological symptoms such as headaches, cognitive difficulties, or even more severe disorders like encephalitis. Ongoing medical follow-up is necessary for addressing these long-term impacts.

Prognosis Based on Early Recognition and Appropriate Management

The prognosis for dengue fever largely depends on the timely detection of symptoms and appropriate therapy of the disease. Early diagnosis and intervention are crucial in preventing serious consequences and improving outcomes.

Early Recognition: Recognizing the early signs and symptoms of dengue fever, such as high fever, severe headache, retro-orbital pain, and rash, allows for rapid medical intervention and supportive care. Early recognition of warning signals for severe dengue, such as stomach pain, recurrent vomiting, and blood, is especially critical.

Appropriate Management: Implementing appropriate management measures, including hydration therapy, pain relief, and monitoring for complications, greatly improves patient outcomes. Following established treatment recommendations and protocols ensures that patients receive the appropriate attention and interventions.

Surveillance and Follow-Up: Continuous monitoring and follow-up during the critical phase of dengue fever are necessary. This includes routine examination of vital signs, analytical measurements, and clinical symptoms to detect any deterioration or problems early.

Role of Healthcare Professionals in Treatment

Healthcare professionals play a critical role in the proper treatment and management of dengue fever. Their tasks encompass diagnosis, patient education, supportive treatment, and monitoring for problems.

Diagnosis: Accurate and quick diagnosis is the first step in controlling dengue fever. Healthcare providers must be proficient at recognizing clinical signs and symptoms and applying relevant laboratory testing to establish the diagnosis.

Patient Education: Educating patients and caregivers about dengue fever, its transmission, and preventive actions is critical. This includes guidance on preventing mosquito bites, recognizing warning signals, and understanding the necessity of water and effective medicine administration.

Supportive Care: Providing supportive care, such as hydration management and pain alleviation, is a cornerstone of dengue treatment. Healthcare practitioners must ensure that patients receive adequate fluids, suitable medications, and required interventions to manage symptoms appropriately.

Monitoring for Complications: Vigilant monitoring for complications, such as hemorrhage, shock, and organ involvement, is important. Healthcare workers must be taught to spot early indicators of deterioration and respond immediately to avert disastrous outcomes.

Interdisciplinary Collaboration: Managing dengue fever often needs collaboration among multiple healthcare professions, including physicians, nurses, laboratory technicians, and pharmacists. Effective communication and teamwork enable comprehensive care and better patient outcomes.

Public Health Initiatives: Healthcare professionals also play a part in public health initiatives aimed at controlling and avoiding dengue epidemics. This involves participation in surveillance programs, vector control activities, and community education campaigns.

The management and treatment of dengue fever involve a multi-faceted approach that involves early recognition, appropriate supportive care, and continuous monitoring for complications. Healthcare workers play a crucial role in delivering care, educating patients, and contributing to public health efforts to manage and prevent dengue outbreaks. Through a combination of good medical therapy and public health interventions, the impact of dengue fever on affected populations can be reduced, and patient outcomes can be greatly improved.

Chapter 6

Prevention Strategies

Preventing dengue illness needs a multimodal approach that targets the mosquito vectors, lowers human-mosquito interaction, and promotes community knowledge. These techniques are critical for preventing the spread of dengue and maintaining public health. Here are some thorough techniques to prevent dengue fever:

How to Fight This Deadly Disease

Dengue fever, caused by the dengue virus transmitted through mosquito bites, can be effectively combated through a mix of personal and community-level efforts. To battle this dangerous disease, it is vital to understand the channels of transmission, adopt preventive measures, and seek appropriate medical care when necessary. Here are specific steps to combat dengue fever:

Personal Protection Measures

Repellents

Using insect repellents is one of the most effective strategies to avoid mosquito bites and lower the risk of dengue fever. Repellents containing DEET, picaridin, IR3535, or oil of lemon eucalyptus are recommended for their potency. When applying repellant, it is vital to follow the following guidelines:

Application: Apply repellant to exposed skin and clothing. Reapply as instructed on the product label, especially after sweating or washing.

Safety: Choose a repellant suitable for your age range and follow the usage instructions. For youngsters, use products specifically intended for them and avoid applying repellent on their hands or near their eyes and lips.

Combination with Sunscreen: If using both sunscreen and repellant, apply the sunscreen, allow it to dry, and then apply the repellent.

Clothing

Wearing suitable attire is another vital measure to prevent mosquito bites. Here are some tips:

Long-Sleeved Shirts and Pants: Wear long-sleeved shirts and long pants to cover as much skin as possible. Light-colored clothing is preferable as it is less enticing to mosquitoes.

Permethrin-Treated Clothing: Treating clothing and gear with permethrin, an insect repellent, gives further protection. Permethrin-treated clothes stay effective even after several washes.

Avoiding Dark Colors: Mosquitoes are attracted to dark colors, so wearing light-colored clothing can help decrease bites.

Vector Control Measures: Mosquito Prevention and Eradication

Controlling the mosquito population is crucial in preventing dengue disease. Effective vector management strategies focus on limiting mosquito breeding areas and minimizing mosquito-human contact. These strategies can be applied at both individual and community levels:

Environmental Management

Eliminate Breeding Sites: Mosquitoes lay their eggs in standing water. Often empty, clean, or cover anything that can gather water, such as flower pots, buckets, bird baths, and abandoned tires. Ensure that water storage containers are closely covered.

Proper Waste Disposal: Dispose of solid waste properly to prevent water collection in discarded containers. Ensure that trash is collected and discarded routinely.

Drainage Systems: Maintain good drainage systems to prevent water stagnation. Clean gutters and drains to ensure water flow freely.

Biological Control

Predators and Larvicides: Introduce natural predators, such as fish that consume mosquito larvae, into water bodies. Use biological larvicides like Bacillus thuringiensis israelensis (Bti) to target mosquito larvae in water containers.

Genetic Control: Research and apply genetic control strategies, such as releasing genetically modified mosquitoes that are sterile or carry deadly genes to reduce mosquito populations.

Chemical Control

pesticides: Use pesticides to kill adult mosquitoes and larvae. Apply pesticide sprays or fogging in high-risk areas, especially during epidemics. Ensure correct usage of insecticides to avoid resistance development.

Larvicides: Apply larvicides to water bodies that cannot be drained or covered. These compounds inhibit mosquito larvae from maturing into adults.

Community Engagement and Education

Community involvement is vital for the efficacy of vector control efforts. Educating the population about dengue prevention and promoting active participation in mosquito control activities can dramatically reduce the risk of dengue transmission:

Public Awareness programs: Conduct educational programs to teach the public about dengue transmission, symptoms, and preventative options. Use multiple media outlets, such as TV, radio, social media, and community activities, to reach a wide audience.

Community Clean-Up Programs: Organize community clean-up programs to eliminate mosquito breeding areas. Encourage people to participate in regular cleaning and maintenance tasks.

School Programs: Implement dengue education programs in schools to teach youngsters about the need for mosquito control and personal protection measures.

What you can do if you get dengue fever

In late June, the Centers for Disease Control and Prevention (CDC) issued a warning about the elevated risk of dengue illnesses in the United States. Dengue, spread by the same mosquitoes that give Zika and chikungunya, is witnessing a boom across the Americas, partially due to climate change. The US is not immune to this epidemic, although identifying dengue can be tricky. Mild cases frequently resemble other fever-causing infections, and many American doctors may not routinely screen for dengue.

Recognizing Dengue Symptoms

To better equip yourself in diagnosing dengue, be proactive with your healthcare providers. If you reside in or have traveled to places where dengue is endemic, notify your doctor. Nearly half the world's population resides in places at risk for dengue.

Dengue Fever in the US

While global dengue cases are growing, only approximately 25% of infected persons feel ill. For those affected, symptoms might be severe. Known as "breakbone fever," dengue can produce fever, severe headache, muscle and joint pain, skin rashes, and pain behind the eyes. Symptoms normally arise within two weeks of being bitten by an infected mosquito and persist between 2 and 7 days. Most folks recover within a week.

Dengue is conveyed through the bite of an infected female Aedes mosquito and is not communicable like respiratory infections such as COVID-19. If you suspect you have dengue, consult a healthcare provider. Blood tests are necessary for an appropriate diagnosis, with samples sent to state health agencies or commercial labs for processing.

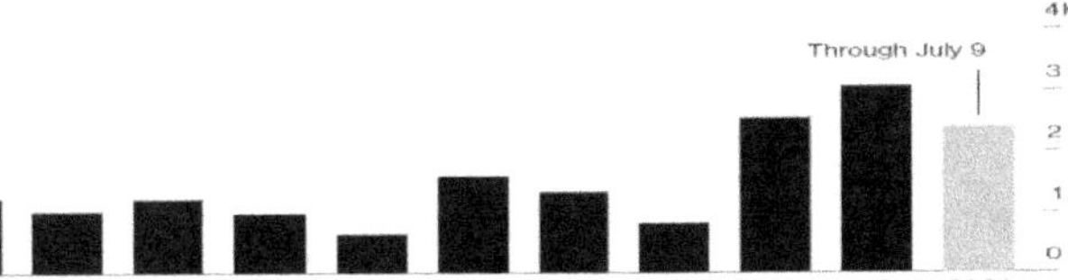

Managing Dengue Symptoms

While awaiting test results, relax, hydrate, and take acetaminophen (Tylenol) for pain relief. Sidestep aspirin or ibuprofen, as these can cause bleeding. Unfortunately, there are no specific therapies for dengue.

Severe dengue, occurring in around 5% of cases, can become life-threatening within hours, leading to shock, internal bleeding, and even death. Emergency symptoms include abdominal discomfort, recurrent vomiting, nose or gum bleeding, vomiting blood, blood in stool, or extreme exhaustion. These indications often develop 24 to 48 hours after the fever passes. If you encounter these symptoms, seek emergency medical assistance immediately.

The CDC is researching new tactics to battle the spike in dengue cases, but you may take preventive precautions. When traveling to dengue-endemic areas, use EPA-registered insect repellents and wear loose, long-sleeved clothing. While a dengue vaccination is not currently licensed for US tourists, other precautions can be beneficial.

If you reside in dengue-prone locations, use window and door screens or bed nets to keep mosquitoes out. If you contract dengue, limit the risk of transferring it to others. During the first week of illness, the virus is present in your blood, and a mosquito bite can transfer it to others.

Staying educated and taking care can help manage and avoid dengue illnesses. The CDC continues to monitor and handle the situation, but personal attention is crucial in countering this rising health concern.

Additional Alert

In a related health advisory, Bloomberg research indicated that some generic erectile dysfunction medications, like Viagra and Cialis, may have been licensed using false data from Synapse Labs in India. The US Food and Medicine Administration (FDA) has warned medicine producers but has not stated which individual drugs are affected, citing confidentiality. This has generated worries among professionals about the necessity for public transparency.

By remaining informed and watchful, you may help protect yourself and others from dengue and stay aware of other vital health alerts.

Long-Term Effects and Post-Dengue Syndrome

While most persons recover totally from dengue infection, some may endure long-term complications, known as post-dengue syndrome. Understanding and regulating these consequences is vital for general health and well-being:

Prolonged Fatigue

Chronic exhaustion: Some persons may feel chronic exhaustion and weakness, which can linger for weeks or months. This post-viral weariness might impair everyday activities and quality of life.

Management: To manage chronic fatigue, it is necessary to get appropriate rest, keep a healthy diet, and engage in light physical activity as tolerated. Consult a healthcare provider if fatigue persists or worsens.

Joint and Muscle Pain

Persistent Pain: Joint and muscular pain, known as arthralgia, might remain following recovery from dengue fever. This discomfort can be excruciating and may require continuing care.

Pain Relief: Over-the-counter pain medications, such as paracetamol, can help control pain. Physical therapy and mild exercises may also bring assistance.

Psychological Effects

Mental Health: The stress of severe disease and the impact on physical health can lead to psychological repercussions, such as depression and anxiety. These impacts should not be neglected and may require mental health treatment.

Therapy: Seek therapy or mental health care if you develop signs of depression or anxiety. Support groups and therapy can help handle these psychological impacts.

Prognosis Based on Early Recognition and Appropriate Management

The prognosis for dengue fever largely hinges on early diagnosis of symptoms and adequate management. Timely action can avert severe consequences and improve outcomes:

Early Recognition

Importance of Early Diagnosis: Recognizing the early signs and symptoms of dengue fever enables rapid medical attention and supportive care. Early identification and treatment can prevent the progression of severe dengue.

Knowledge: Increasing knowledge among the public and healthcare providers about the signs and symptoms of dengue fever is critical for early recognition and response.

Appropriate Management

Supportive Care: Effective management of dengue fever entails providing supportive care to manage symptoms and prevent complications. Hydration, pain treatment, and monitoring for warning indications are critical components of supportive care.

Recommendations: Following established treatment recommendations and procedures ensures that patients receive the proper care and treatments to improve results.

Community Efforts and Public Health Initiatives

Community activities and public health initiatives are vital in the fight against dengue fever. The collective work of communities, along with targeted public health initiatives, can considerably lower the occurrence of this disease. These efforts focus on education, vector control,

and coordination among diverse stakeholders to establish
an environment that minimizes the risk of dengue
transmission.

Public Education Campaigns

Effective public education programs are vital for raising
knowledge about dengue disease and advocating
preventive measures. These efforts aim to inform the
public about the hazards of dengue, its symptoms, and
the activities individuals can take to protect themselves
and their communities.

Awareness Programs: These programs use multiple
media platforms, including television, radio, social
media, and community gatherings, to reach a large
audience. They underline the necessity of eliminating
mosquito breeding areas, utilizing repellents, and getting
medical assistance promptly if symptoms emerge.

School Initiatives: Schools play a serious role in
educating youngsters about dengue prevention.
Educational programs might include interactive sessions,
informational materials, and activities that teach students
about mosquito control and personal protective
measures.

Community Engagement

Community engagement is important to the effectiveness
of dengue prevention measures. Active participation of
community members ensures that preventive actions are
executed successfully and consistently.

Community Clean-Up Efforts: Regular community clean-up efforts help remove mosquito breeding places. These actions involve cleaning public spaces, clearing stagnant water, and properly disposing of waste. Community leaders can organize these drives and encourage mass involvement.

Volunteer Programs: Trained volunteers can educate residents about dengue prevention and aid in monitoring and eradicating mosquito breeding places. These programs develop a sense of ownership and responsibility within the community.

Collaboration with Local Authorities

Collaboration between communities and local government is vital for executing large-scale dengue prevention initiatives. Local governments can provide funding, assistance, and enforcement to ensure the effectiveness of these efforts.

Vector Control Programs: Local authorities can develop vector control programs that involve frequent insecticide spraying, larviciding, and monitoring of mosquito populations. These activities should be coordinated with community efforts to maximize impact.

Legislation and Regulation: Enforcing regulations that limit the accumulation of stagnant water and ensuring adequate waste disposal can reduce mosquito breeding places. Local governments can also apply fines for non-compliance to encourage adherence to these restrictions.

Use of Insect Repellents

Insect repellents are a crucial aid in minimizing mosquito bites and reducing the risk of dengue fever. The appropriate application of repellents can give significant protection against mosquito bites, especially in high-risk settings.

Types of Insect Repellents

Several varieties of insect repellents are available, each with differing degrees of effectiveness. The most commonly used repellents contain active chemicals as DEET, picaridin, IR3535, and oil of lemon eucalyptus.

DEET: DEET is one of the most effective and extensively used insect repellents. It provides long-lasting protection against mosquito bites and is available in various concentrations. Products with 20-30% DEET are generally suitable for most people and children over two months of age.

Picaridin: Picaridin is another powerful repellent that gives protection similar to DEET. It is less oily and has a softer odor, making it a preferable choice for some individuals. Picaridin products are available in various concentrations, often ranging from 10–20%.

IR3535: IR3535 is a synthetic repellent that provides great protection against mosquitoes. It is less irritating to the skin and eyes compared to DEET and picaridin.

IR3535 compounds are available in concentrations up to 20%.

Oil of Lemon Eucalyptus: Oil of lemon eucalyptus is a natural repellent obtained from the lemon eucalyptus tree. It provides protection comparable to low quantities of DEET and is widely used as a natural alternative. Products containing 30% oil of lemon eucalyptus are widely recommended.

Application Guidelines

To enhance the efficiency of insect repellents, it is vital to apply them correctly. Here are some guidelines for proper application:

Apply to Exposed Skin: Apply repellent to all exposed skin, following the package recommendations. Avoid applying repellant to cuts, wounds, or irritated skin.

Avoid Eyes and Mouth: Do not apply repellant near the eyes or mouth. When applying it to the face, spray the repellent into your hands first and then apply it to the face.

Use on garments: Some repellents can be applied to garments for added protection. Follow the package directions to ensure safe and effective use.

Reapply as Needed: Reapply repellant as indicated, especially after sweating, swimming, or washing. The length of protection varies based on the active component and concentration.

Best Practices for Wearing Protective Clothing

Loose-Fitting Clothing: Loose-fitting clothing is less likely to be penetrated by mosquitoes than tight-fitting clothes. Ensure that sleeves and pant legs are not too tight to allow for airflow and comfort.

Layering: In chilly areas or during twilight hours, layering garments can provide further protection. Layering also helps trap body heat and provides an additional barrier against mosquito bites.

Regular Inspection: Regularly inspect clothing for holes or tears that could allow mosquitoes to infiltrate. Repair or replace damaged garments to ensure adequate protection.

Eliminating Breeding Sites

Eliminating mosquito breeding areas is one of the most effective ways to minimize the risk of dengue illness. Mosquitoes lay their eggs in standing water, hence removing or cleaning these breeding places can radically reduce mosquito populations.

Identifying Breeding Sites

Stagnant Water: Mosquitoes breed in stagnant water, thus it is crucial to detect and eradicate sources of standing water surrounding houses and communities. Common breeding locations include flower pots, buckets, bird baths, discarded tires, and clogged gutters.

Water Storage Containers: Water storage containers, such as barrels, tanks, and cisterns, can also serve as breeding sites if not adequately protected. Ensure that these containers are properly well tight up to prevent mosquitoes from laying eggs.

Eliminating and Treating Breeding Sites

Regular Inspection: Conduct regular inspections of your property and neighboring areas to detect and eradicate potential breeding places. Remove, empty, or cover containers that can gather water.

Proper Disposal: Dispose of solid waste properly to prevent water collection in discarded containers. Ensure that trash is collected and discarded routinely.

Larvicides: Use larvicides to remediate water bodies that cannot be emptied or covered. Larvicides, such as Bacillus thuringiensis israelensis (Bti), target mosquito larvae and prevent them from maturing into adults.

Drainage Systems: Maintain good drainage systems to prevent water stagnation. Clean gutters and drains to ensure water flow easily and do not accumulate.

Avoiding Peak Mosquito Hours and Areas

Avoiding peak mosquito hours and places is another excellent method to lower the risk of mosquito bites and dengue fever. Mosquitoes are most active during various times of the day and in specific environments.

Peak Mosquito Hours

Dawn and evening: Mosquitoes, particularly Aedes aegypti, are most active during dawn and evening. During these periods, it is vital to take extra steps to avoid mosquito bites.

Nighttime: While Aedes mosquitoes usually bite during the day, some species are active at night. Using bed nets and other preventative measures can help lower the danger of overnight bites.

High-Risk Areas

Shady regions: Mosquitoes usually rest in shady regions all through the day. Avoid spending time in shady, humid settings where mosquitoes are likely to be present.

Vegetation: Areas with lush vegetation, such as forests, gardens, and parks, can host mosquitoes. Take precautions, such as wearing protective clothing and utilizing repellents, when visiting these locations.

Best Practices for Avoiding Mosquito Bites

Stay Indoors: During peak mosquito activity times, stay indoors as much as possible. Use screens on windows and doors to keep this mosquitoes out.

Use Bed Nets: When sleeping, especially in locations where mosquitoes are widespread, use bed nets sprayed with insecticide. Bed nets provide a physical barrier and additional protection against mosquito bites.

Air Conditioning: Use air conditioning, if available, to keep indoor rooms cool and mosquito-free. Mosquitoes are less likely to thrive in cooler, air-conditioned areas.

Integrated Approaches for Dengue Prevention

Effective dengue prevention involves an integrated approach that combines personal protection measures, community activities, and public health initiatives. By implementing a comprehensive plan, people and communities can dramatically minimize the risk of dengue transmission and preserve public health.

Coordination and Collaboration

Multisectoral Collaboration: Effective dengue prevention needs collaboration among multiple sectors, including health, education, environmental management, and local government. Coordinated efforts ensure the implementation of comprehensive initiatives and maximize their impact.

Community Involvement: Engaging communities in dengue prevention activities is vital for success. Community members play a critical role in locating and eliminating breeding locations, advocating personal safety measures, and engaging in public health programs.

Continuous Monitoring and Evaluation

Surveillance Systems: Robust surveillance systems are necessary for monitoring dengue spread and recognizing outbreaks. Timely data collection and analysis enable public health officials to respond swiftly and effectively to emerging hazards.

Evaluation of programs: Regular evaluation of dengue prevention programs aids assess their efficiency and identifies areas for improvement. Continuous monitoring and review guarantee that strategies stay relevant and impactful.

Community activities and public health initiatives are vital in the fight against dengue fever. The collective work of communities, along with targeted public health initiatives, can considerably lower the occurrence of this disease. These efforts focus on education, vector control, and coordination among diverse stakeholders to establish an environment that minimizes the risk of dengue transmission.

Public Education Campaigns

Effective public education programs are vital for raising knowledge about dengue disease and advocating preventive measures. These efforts aim to inform the public about the hazards of dengue, its symptoms, and the activities individuals can take to protect themselves and their communities.

Awareness Programs: These programs use multiple media platforms, including television, radio, social media, and community gatherings, to reach a large audience. They underline the necessity of eliminating mosquito breeding areas, utilizing repellents, and getting medical assistance promptly if symptoms emerge.

Community Engagement

Community engagement is important to the effectiveness of dengue prevention measures. Active participation of community members ensures that preventive actions are executed successfully and consistently.

Community Clean-Up Efforts: Regular community clean-up efforts help remove mosquito breeding places. These actions involve cleaning public spaces, clearing stagnant water, and properly disposing of waste. Community leaders can organize these drives and encourage mass involvement.

Volunteer Programs: Trained volunteers can educate residents about dengue prevention and aid in monitoring and eradicating mosquito breeding places. These programs develop a sense of ownership and responsibility within the community.

Collaboration with Local Authorities

Collaboration between communities and local government is vital for executing large-scale dengue prevention initiatives. Local governments can provide funding, assistance, and enforcement to ensure the effectiveness of these efforts.

Vector Control Programs: Local authorities can develop vector control programs that involve frequent insecticide spraying, larviciding, and monitoring of mosquito populations. These activities should be coordinated with community efforts to maximize impact.

Legislation and Regulation: Enforcing regulations that limit the accumulation of stagnant water and ensuring adequate waste disposal can reduce mosquito breeding places. Local governments can also apply fines for non-compliance to encourage adherence to these restrictions.

Application Guidelines

To enhance the efficiency of insect repellents, it is vital to apply them correctly. Here are some guidelines for proper application:

Apply to Exposed Skin: Apply repellent to all exposed skin, following the package recommendations. Avoid applying repellant to cuts, wounds, or irritated skin.

Reapply as Needed: Reapply repellant as indicated, especially after sweating, swimming, or washing. The length of protection varies based on the active component and concentration.

Dengue Vaccine: Available Options and Limitations

Vaccination is a vital component in the fight against dengue fever, delivering a preventive intervention that can greatly lower the frequency and severity of the disease. However, the development and distribution of dengue vaccines have faced several hurdles, resulting in a restricted number of choices currently accessible.

Available Dengue Vaccines

The first dengue vaccine to be licensed for use was Dengvaxia, manufactured by Sanofi Pasteur. Other vaccinations are in varying phases of development, but dengue fever remains the most widely discussed and examined.

Dengvaxia (CYD-TDV): Dengvaxia is a live attenuated tetravalent dengue vaccine that targets all four dengue virus serotypes (DENV-1 to DENV-4). It was originally approved for use in numerous countries in 2015. This vaccination was provided in a three-dose schedule over 12 months.

Efficacy and Safety

The efficacy and safety of Dengvaxia have been the subject of much research and discussion. Clinical trials have demonstrated that the vaccination gives various amounts of protection against the different serotypes and age groups.

Efficacy by Serotype: Dengvaxia has proven stronger efficacy against some serotypes (e.g., DENV-3 and DENV-4) compared to others (e.g., DENV-1 and DENV-2). The vaccine's overall effectiveness is predicted to be around 60–80% for people with prior dengue illness.

Age-Dependent Efficacy: Studies have revealed that vaccination is more effective in older children and adolescents, particularly those aged 9-16 years. Younger children, especially those under the age of 9, have exhibited lesser efficacy and a higher risk of catastrophic outcomes if they get dengue following vaccination.

Limitations and Concerns

While Dengvaxia represents a substantial development in dengue prevention, its usage is accompanied by various restrictions and concerns.

Risk of Severe Dengue: One of the major concerns with Dengvaxia is the increased risk of severe dengue in seronegative persons (those who have never been infected with dengue previously). This paradoxical effect occurs because the vaccination simulates a first infection, and subsequent natural infection can lead to a significant immune response.

Pre-Vaccination Screening: Due to the risk of severe dengue in seronegative persons, the World Health Organization (WHO) recommends pre-vaccination screening to determine an individual's serostatus. Only patients with a prior dengue illness should receive the vaccine, which limits its widespread use and creates logistical obstacles.

Limited Duration of Protection: The protection afforded by Dengvaxia is not lifelong. Studies reveal that the vaccine provides effective protection for around 4-5 years, after which the immunity wanes. This demands further investigation into booster doses or alternate immunization procedures.

Ongoing Research and Future Prospects

The development of dengue vaccines continues to be an important area of study, with multiple candidates at various stages of clinical trials. These projects aim to address the shortcomings of Dengvaxia and create safer and more effective solutions.

TAK-003 (Takeda Vaccine): TAK-003, created by Takeda Pharmaceutical Company, is a tetravalent live attenuated vaccine. Early clinical trials have shown excellent results, with good efficacy across all four serotypes and an acceptable safety profile. The vaccine is now undergoing phase III testing.

TV003/TV005 (National Institutes of Health): The TV003/TV005 vaccine candidate, developed by the National Institutes of Health (NIH), is another intriguing possibility. It is a live-attenuated tetravalent vaccination that has shown excellent levels of protection in early studies. It is currently being investigated in larger trials.

Travel Advisories and Precautions in Endemic Areas

Traveling to dengue-endemic areas carries a risk of catching the disease, making it vital for tourists to take appropriate precautions. Public health authorities, like the Centers for Disease Control and Prevention (CDC) and the World Health Organization (WHO), issue travel advisories and provide suggestions to help tourists minimize their risk.

Pre-Travel Preparations

Before traveling to a dengue-endemic location, people should take numerous precautions to prepare and protect themselves.

Visit healthcare practitioners: Travelers should visit with healthcare practitioners or travel medicine specialists to receive specific advice based on their destination and health state. This consultation can include discussions regarding immunizations, preventive measures, and what to do if symptoms of dengue arise.

Immunization Considerations: While Dengvaxia is not indicated for travelers without a history of dengue infection, those with a confirmed past infection may consider immunization choices with their healthcare physician. Ongoing research and the potential approval of new vaccinations may broaden the options accessible to travelers in the future.

Travel Insurance: Purchasing comprehensive travel insurance that covers medical expenses, including the cost of treatment for dengue fever, is advisable. This assures that passengers have access to vital medical care if they become ill during their trip.

Precautionary Measures During Travel

During travel to dengue-endemic areas, people should adhere to certain preventative steps to limit their risk of mosquito bites and dengue infection.

Use of Insect Repellents: Applying insect repellents containing DEET, picaridin, or oil of lemon eucalyptus to exposed skin is vital. These repellents give strong protection against mosquito bites and should be reapplied as advised, especially after sweating or swimming.

Staying in Mosquito-Protected lodgings: Travelers should seek lodgings with air conditioning, window and door screens, or mosquito nets to prevent mosquito ingress. Using bed nets when sleeping, especially in locations without air conditioning, can significantly lower the danger of bites.

Avoiding Peak Mosquito Activity: Mosquitoes that spread dengue are most active during the early morning and late afternoon. Travelers should minimize outdoor activity during these peak periods or take extra precautions if they must be outside.

Post-Travel Considerations

After returning from a dengue-endemic location, travelers should continue to check their health and take appropriate precautions if symptoms arise.

Monitoring for Symptoms: Dengue symptoms might show up to 14 days after returning from an infected location. Travelers should remain watchful and seek medical assistance if they experience any signs of dengue fever.

Preventing Local Transmission: If a traveler is diagnosed with dengue fever, they should make efforts to prevent local mosquito bites to avoid passing the virus to mosquitoes that could infect others. This involves applying insect repellents, wearing protective clothing, and staying indoors as much as possible.

Importance of Public Health Measures

Travel advisories and public health initiatives play a key role in avoiding the spread of dengue disease. Travelers should be aware of current cautions and follow advised recommendations to protect themselves and others.

Monitoring Outbreaks: Public health agencies regularly monitor dengue outbreaks and offer current information and travel advisories. Travelers should check for the latest advisories before arranging their travel and be informed about the dengue condition in their location.

Dengue fever poses a serious global health concern, particularly in endemic locations where the risk of infection is high. While the development of dengue vaccines offers hope for reducing the occurrence of the disease, current choices like Dengvaxia come with restrictions and require careful thought and pre-vaccination screening. Ongoing research into novel vaccinations holds hope for more effective and safer choices in the future.

For travelers to dengue-endemic areas, taking preventive steps is vital. This involves visiting healthcare providers, applying insect repellents, wearing protective clothes, staying in mosquito-protected lodgings, and recognizing and responding to symptoms promptly. Public health programs and travel advisories give guidance and support to limit the risk of dengue infection and shield public health.

Through a combination of vaccines, personal preventive measures, and community participation, the global burden of dengue fever can be minimized, safeguarding the health and well-being of individuals and communities worldwide.

Chapter 7

Research and Future Directions

The fight against dengue fever continues to fuel considerable research efforts globally, concentrating on understanding the virus, generating viable vaccines, and enhancing epidemiological control methods. This continuous study is crucial for tackling the chronic and evolving threat posed by dengue disease.

Recent Advancements in Dengue Research

Recent developments in dengue research have advanced our understanding of the virus, its transmission patterns, and its impact on human health. These advancements span various fields, including virology, immunology, and epidemiology.

1. Virological Research:

Genomic Sequencing: Advances in genomic sequencing have revealed detailed insights into the genetic makeup of dengue viruses. This information is vital for following the evolution of different serotypes and understanding their transmission patterns.

Virus-Host Interactions: Research has highlighted the complicated interactions between the dengue virus and host cells. This involves studying how the virus evades the immune system and the strategies it uses to proliferate within host cells.

Viral Proteins: Studies on viral proteins, such as the envelope (E) and non-structural (NS) proteins, have shown their functions in the virus's life cycle and pathogenicity. This understanding is critical for designing targeted antiviral treatments.

2. Immunological Research:

Immune Response Mechanisms: Investigations investigating how the human immune system responds to dengue infection have revealed critical immune cells and chemicals involved in the response. This consist of the role of T cells, B cells, and cytokines in managing the infection.

Antibody-Dependent Enhancement (ADE): Understanding ADE, a phenomenon where pre-existing antibodies from a previous dengue infection might worsen the severity of a subsequent illness, has been a key emphasis. This research is vital for generating safe and effective vaccinations.

Cross-Protection: Studies have studied the potential for cross-protection between various dengue serotypes. This includes exploring how immunity to one serotype can influence the response to another serotype.

3. Epidemiological Research:

Disease Burden Estimation: Research has improved estimates of the worldwide burden of dengue, highlighting places with the highest incidence and identifying risk factors for severe disease.

Transmission Dynamics: Studies on the dynamics of dengue transmission have revealed insights into how environmental factors, such as climate change and urbanization, influence the spread of the virus.

Mathematical Modeling: Mathematical models have been built to anticipate dengue outbreaks and assess the impact of various control methods. These models are essential instruments for public health planning and action.

Vaccine Development Progress and Challenges

The development of dengue vaccines has been a major focus of study, given the huge potential for reducing the incidence and severity of the disease. Despite great improvement, some challenges remain.

1. Dengvaxia:

Efficacy and Safety: Dengvaxia, the first licensed dengue vaccine, has exhibited varying efficacy across different age groups and serotypes. While it protects those with a prior dengue infection, it raises a risk of severe sickness in seronegative individuals.

Pre-Vaccination Screening: The requirement for pre-vaccination screening to determine serostatus has hampered the broad usage of Dengvaxia. This adds complexity to immunization efforts and raises logistical issues in resource-limited areas.

2. New Vaccine Candidates:

TAK-003 (Takeda Vaccine): TAK-003 has shown promising results in clinical studies, with strong efficacy across all four serotypes and an acceptable safety profile. Ongoing phase III trials are expected to offer more definitive data on its effectiveness and long-term protection.

TV003/TV005 (NIH Vaccine): TV003/TV005 is another potential candidate, displaying high levels of protection in early trials. Research is ongoing to examine its efficacy and safety in wider populations.

3. Challenges in Vaccine Development:

Heterogeneity of Dengue Viruses: The genetic variety of dengue viruses and the presence of four unique serotypes provide considerable obstacles to vaccine development. A successful vaccine must give balanced protection against all serotypes.

Risk of ADE: The risk of ADE complicates vaccine development, as vaccinations must avoid enhancing the severity of the following diseases. This needs a detailed understanding of immune responses and careful creation of vaccination formulations.

Long-Term Protection: Ensuring long-term protection against dengue is another difficulty. Current vaccinations protect a limited term, necessitating research into booster dosages and other vaccination procedures.

Emerging Trends in Dengue Epidemiology and Control

Dengue epidemiology and management measures are always evolving, affected by new study discoveries, technology breakthroughs, and changing environmental and societal factors.

1. Climate Change and Urbanization:

Impact of Climate Change: Climate change has a major impact on dengue transmission. Rising temperatures, increased rainfall, and variations in humidity produce favorable circumstances for the multiplication of Aedes mosquitoes, the major carriers of dengue.

Urbanization: Rapid urbanization, particularly in poorer nations, contributes to the spread of dengue. Urban settings provide perfect breeding habitats for mosquitoes, such as stagnant water in containers, and promote human-mosquito contact.

2. Vector Control Innovations:

Wolbachia-Infected Mosquitoes: The release of mosquitoes infected with Wolbachia, a bacterium that inhibits the ability of mosquitoes to spread dengue, is a promising vector control strategy. Field investigations have demonstrated substantial reductions in dengue transmission in regions where Wolbachia-infected mosquitoes have been released.

Genetically Modified Mosquitoes: Genetic engineering techniques are being utilized to generate mosquitoes that are either sterile or less capable of transmitting dengue. These genetically modified mosquitoes are released into the environment to lower the mosquito population and stop the transmission cycle.

3. Surveillance and Early Warning Systems:

Enhanced Surveillance Systems: Advances in technology have enhanced dengue surveillance systems. Real-time data gathering, geographic information systems (GIS), and remote sensing capabilities enable more accurate surveillance of dengue outbreaks and identification of high-risk locations.

Early Warning Systems: Early warning systems that use climate and environmental data to predict dengue outbreaks are being developed. These systems enable for prompt public health actions and resource allocation to prevent or minimize outbreaks.

4. Community Engagement and Education:

Community Involvement: Engaging communities in dengue control activities is vital for success. Public health initiatives that educate communities about dengue prevention, mosquito control, and the significance of early medical intervention can greatly lower the illness burden.

Behavioral Interventions: Research into behavioral interventions tries to understand and improve human behaviors that contribute to dengue transmission. This involves promoting the use of insect repellents, proper waste disposal, and eliminating mosquito breeding areas.

5. Integrated Disease Management:

Intersectoral Collaboration: Effective dengue control involves collaboration across different sectors, including health, environment, education, and local government. Integrated disease management approaches that incorporate different stakeholders are necessary for thorough and sustainable control efforts.

Holistic Strategies: Combining vector control, vaccination, public education, and robust surveillance systems creates a holistic approach to dengue management. This multi-faceted technique addresses the complexity of dengue transmission and enhances the overall effectiveness of control measures.

Research and future directions in dengue control are crucial for tackling the continuous threat of this illness. Recent discoveries in virology, immunology, and epidemiology have increased our understanding of dengue and guided the creation of innovative control methods. While obstacles remain, particularly in vaccine development, ongoing research gives hope for more effective and safer alternatives. Emerging developments in vector management, surveillance, and community participation underscore the dynamic character of dengue epidemiology and the need for adaptable and integrated interventions. Through continuous research and collaboration, great progress may be made in lowering the worldwide burden of dengue fever and protecting vulnerable populations.

Chapter 8

Living with Dengue

Living with dengue fever poses a unique set of obstacles for people impacted by the disease, demanding both physical and mental strength. The experience of dealing with dengue fever extends beyond the acute health concerns, impacting the psychological well-being and daily life of individuals and communities. Understanding how to live with the sickness, its psychological implications, and the tales of those impacted can provide vital insights for managing and overcoming this devastating illness.

Coping Strategies During Dengue Outbreak

Dengue outbreaks can cause major disturbances to ordinary life, needing strong coping mechanisms to handle the disease and its repercussions. Here are some ideas to help individuals and communities overcome these hard times:

1. Staying Informed:

Accurate Information: Access to credible information regarding dengue, its symptoms, treatment, and prevention is vital. Understanding the disease helps individuals make informed decisions about their health and take necessary preventive steps.

Public Health Updates: Keeping up with public health advisories and updates can help folks be aware of the current situation, including outbreak locations and recommended safeguards.

2. Personal Health Management:

Rest and Hydration: Dengue fever generally causes significant weariness and dehydration. Ensuring enough rest and being hydrated is key for healing. Drinking enough water helps to maintain hydration levels and aids the body's healing process.

Pain Management: Managing pain and fever with suitable drugs, as indicated by healthcare specialists, helps alleviate discomfort. Avoiding aspirin and non-steroidal anti-inflammatory medicines (NSAIDs) is recommended due to the danger of bleeding problems.

Monitoring Symptoms: Keeping a close check on symptoms and obtaining medical attention if they worsen is crucial. Early intervention can prevent problems and ensure prompt treatment.

3. Support Networks:

Family and Friends: Leaning on family and friends for emotional and practical support can make a major impact. Loved ones can aid with daily duties, provide companionship, and offer encouragement during the rehabilitation process.

Community Support: Community support groups and organizations can offer resources and assistance. These groups generally provide information, emotional support, and help in accessing medical care.

4. Preventive Measures:

Mosquito Control: Taking action to decrease mosquito exposure is crucial. This involves using mosquito nets, and repellents, and wearing protective clothing to minimize bites.

Environmental Management: Eliminating possible mosquito breeding places, such as standing water in containers, might lower the likelihood of mosquito proliferation and eventual dengue transmission.

Psychological Impacts and Community Resilience

The psychological impact of dengue fever can be severe, impacting not only those who suffer the disease but also their families and communities. Building resilience at both the individual and community levels is vital for coping with the mental health issues brought on by dengue outbreaks.

1. Emotional Distress:

Concern and Anxiety: The uncertainty and concern associated with dengue fever can lead to substantial anxiety. Concerns about health, potential consequences, and the possibility of transferring the disease to loved ones can be overwhelming.

Depression: Prolonged illness and the physical toll of dengue fever can lead to feelings of depression. The loss of normalcy, coupled with physical suffering, might damage emotional well-being.

2. Community Impact:

Social Stigma: In some societies, individuals with dengue fever may endure social stigma and isolation. Misunderstandings about the disease and fear of infection can lead to discrimination and exclusion.

Economic Strain: The economic impact of dengue outbreaks can be severe. Families may suffer financial challenges due to medical bills and lost income from time off work, aggravating stress and worry.

3. Building Resilience:

Mental Health Support: Access to mental health resources, such as counseling and support groups, can help patients cope with the psychological repercussions of dengue fever. Professional support can provide ways to manage anxiety, despair, and stress.

Community Engagement: Strengthening community relationships and fostering a sense of solidarity can help resilience. Community programs that promote knowledge, prevention, and support can lessen the impact of dengue outbreaks.

Education and Empowerment: Empowering folks with knowledge about dengue fever and prevention strategies can develop confidence and reduce fear. Education initiatives that increase awareness and refute falsehoods can lessen stigma and stimulate collaborative action.

Stories of Individuals Affected by Dengue Fever

The personal experiences of persons impacted by dengue fever illustrate the human side of the disease, illustrating the struggles and accomplishments of living with and surviving dengue.

1. Maria's Story: Maria, a mother of three from Brazil, suffered dengue fever during an outbreak in her neighborhood. She recalls the abrupt onset of high temperature, intense joint pain, and crippling tiredness. As a primary caregiver, Maria tried to juggle her responsibilities while battling the illness. Her community gave important support, helping with childcare and domestic duties. Maria's experience underlines the need for community support networks in managing the human burden of dengue illness.

2. Ahmed's Story: Ahmed, a young professional from Pakistan, experienced a serious case of dengue hemorrhagic fever. His condition necessitated hospitalization and careful medical treatment. Ahmed recalls the physical discomfort and mental distress of being separated from his family throughout treatment. The healthcare team's kindness and skill were important in his recuperation. Ahmed's tale shows the essential role of healthcare workers in giving not just medical treatment but also emotional support to patients.

3. Lina's Story: Lina, a college student in the Philippines, acquired dengue illness during her final examinations. The timing adds great stress to an already tough situation. Despite her illness, Lina's ambition to complete her education kept her motivated. Her professors and classmates offered flexibility and support, allowing her to heal without compromising her academic ambitions. Lina's perseverance and the support she received illustrate how academic institutions may play a role in aiding students afflicted by dengue.

4. Carlos's Story: Carlos, a farmer in Mexico, faced many dengue infections throughout the years. His narrative emphasizes the continued threat of dengue in endemic areas and the necessity for continuous vigilance. Carlos's proactive approach to mosquito management on his farm, including utilizing insecticides and eliminating breeding areas, helped safeguard his family and neighborhood. His efforts highlight the impact of individual and community activities in reducing the danger of dengue transmission.

5. Ananya's Story: Ananya, a schoolteacher in India, developed dengue fever during a local outbreak. She highlights the need for early detection of symptoms and obtaining urgent medical assistance. Ananya's experience with dengue fever led her to educate her kids and their families about the disease. Her efforts to increase awareness and encourage preventive measures underscore the vital importance of education in combatting dengue.

Coping with Dengue in Everyday Life

Living with dengue fever demands a diversified approach to cope with the physical, mental, and social obstacles provided by the condition. Here are more techniques to manage the impact of dengue fever in daily life:

1. Physical Care:

Balanced Diet: Maintaining a balanced diet helps strengthen the immune system and aid recuperation. Consuming a variety of fruits, vegetables, and proteins helps give the vital nutrients for recovery.

Gentle Exercise: Engaging in modest physical activity, as tolerated, helps improve circulation and boost general well-being. Gentle stretching or walking might help reduce stiffness and enhance mood.

Hygiene Practices: Practicing excellent hygiene, such as regular handwashing and keeping living places clean, can avoid subsequent infections and provide a healthy environment.

2. Emotional Support:

Mindfulness and Relaxation: Techniques such as mindfulness, meditation, and deep breathing exercises can assist manage stress and anxiety. These routines induce relaxation and increase mental clarity.

Journaling: Keeping a journal to capture thoughts and feelings can provide an outlet for emotional expression and contemplation. It can also help track symptoms and progress during rehabilitation.

Connecting with Others: Maintaining social relationships through phone calls, video chats, or socially distanced visits can provide emotional support and lessen feelings of loneliness.

3. Practical Assistance:

Home Care Support: Enlisting support from family members, friends, or community organizations for duties such as grocery shopping, meal preparation, and childcare helps reduce the load of everyday responsibilities.

Financial Planning: Exploring financial aid programs, insurance choices, and community resources can help manage medical bills and alleviate economic strain.

Accessing Healthcare: Utilizing telehealth services and internet resources can facilitate access to medical care and guidance without the need for regular in-person visits.

Living with dengue fever is a hard experience that requires comprehensive solutions for coping with the sickness and its larger implications. Personal health management, emotional support, and community resilience are critical components of good coping. The experiences of persons affected by dengue fever illustrate the human side of the disease, underlining the significance of support networks, education, and proactive steps in treating and overcoming dengue. By understanding and tackling the various obstacles of living with dengue fever, individuals and communities can strengthen their resilience and improve their overall well-being.

Chapter 9

Dengue Fever in Vulnerable Populations

Individuals who are immunocompromised, children, pregnant women, older people, and people who have comorbidities are among the vulnerable categories who face considerable hurdles when it comes to dengue fever. Since these populations are more likely to experience severe consequences and problems as a result of dengue infection, it is essential to have a thorough understanding of their particular requirements and dangers. It is necessary to take individualized approaches to the prevention, diagnosis, and care of these vulnerable populations to safeguard and support them successfully.

Children

Children are especially prone to dengue fever, and their bodies are smaller and their immune systems are still developing can make them more susceptible to severe forms of the disease. When it comes to children, dengue fever can have various effects, including particular clinical manifestations, complications, and the requirement for specific medical attention.

When it comes to children, clinical presentation:

Symptom Variation: When compared to adults, children may display a very distinct set of symptoms. Indications that are frequently seen in youngsters include a high fever, rash, headache, soreness in the muscles and joints, and indications of vomiting. There are a few non-specific symptoms that infants may exhibit, including irritability, unwillingness to eat, and lethargy.

Severity: Children are at a higher risk of getting severe dengue, including dengue hemorrhagic fever (DHF) and dengue shock syndrome (DSS). It is possible for these illnesses to swiftly advance to stages that are life-threatening if they are not addressed promptly.

Complications and Management:

Fluid Management: Managing fluid balance in children with dengue is critical. Dehydration from high fever and vomiting can be severe, and careful monitoring of fluid intake and output is important to prevent shock.

Bleeding Risks: Children with severe dengue may have bleeding issues. Platelet count monitoring and supportive care to manage bleeding risks are crucial.

Hospitalization: Hospitalization is often essential for children with severe symptoms to ensure careful observation and timely action. Pediatric care personnel are educated to meet the special needs of children with dengue.

Pregnant Women

Pregnant women confront special obstacles when coping with dengue fever, as the sickness can harm both the mother and the growing fetus. Pregnancy changes the immunological response and physiological factors, raising the likelihood of severe outcomes and problems.

Risks and Complications:

Maternal Health: Pregnant women with dengue fever are at higher risk for severe disease, including hemorrhagic complications and pre-eclampsia-like syndrome. These diseases can risk the health of both the mother and the fetus.

Fetal Health: Dengue infection during pregnancy can lead to severe fetal outcomes, including preterm birth, low birth weight, and stillbirth. Vertical transmission of the virus from mother to fetus is also a risk.

Labor & Delivery: Dengue fever near the time of delivery can complicate labor and delivery, increasing the risk of bleeding and necessitating cautious obstetric supervision.

Management Strategies:

Prenatal Care: Pregnant women in dengue-endemic areas should undergo frequent prenatal care to check their health and detect early signs of dengue illness. Education on preventive actions is vital.

Early Diagnosis: Rapid and correct diagnosis of dengue in pregnant women is crucial. Early action can decrease hazards and enhance outcomes.

Multidisciplinary Approach: Managing dengue in pregnant women involves a multidisciplinary team, including obstetricians, infectious disease specialists, and neonatologists, to offer comprehensive treatment for both mother and baby.

Older Adults

Older people, particularly those with underlying health issues, are more susceptible to severe dengue and its consequences. Age-related alterations in the immune system and the presence of comorbidities can increase the disease's impact.

Clinical Challenges:

Comorbidities: Older people commonly have chronic illnesses such as diabetes, hypertension, and cardiovascular disease, which might complicate the management of dengue fever. These disorders raise the likelihood of severe disease and catastrophic outcomes.

Atypical Presentation: Dengue fever in older persons may show atypically, with symptoms such as disorientation, weakness, and restricted mobility, which might be confused with other disorders.

Severe Disease: The probability of developing severe dengue, including DHF and DSS, is increased in older persons. The disease's course can be rapid, requiring attentive monitoring and timely treatment.

Management Considerations:

Comprehensive Care: Managing dengue in older people involves a holistic strategy that tackles both the acute infection and any underlying health issues. Coordination between primary care doctors and specialists is vital.

Supportive Measures: Providing enough hydration, reducing discomfort, and monitoring for indicators of severe disease are critical parts of care. Adjusting medications for comorbidities to prevent interactions and problems is also crucial.

Vaccination: In places where dengue is endemic, older people should be considered for dengue vaccination, if suitable, to lower the risk of infection.

Comorbidities and Immunocompromised Individuals

Individuals with comorbidities and those who are immunocompromised face heightened risks when infected with dengue fever. Their compromised immune systems and other health issues complicate the disease's care and raise the chance of severe results.

Impact of Comorbidities:

Diabetes and Hypertension: Conditions such as diabetes and hypertension might aggravate the severity of dengue fever. These comorbidities are related to increased vascular permeability and higher risks of bleeding and shock.

Chronic Kidney Disease: Individuals with chronic kidney disease may face heightened symptoms and problems due to reduced renal function and fluid balance concerns.

Cardiovascular Disease: Dengue fever can stress the cardiovascular system, leading to consequences such as myocarditis and the worsening of previous cardiac problems.

Immunocompromised Individuals:

HIV/AIDS: People living with HIV/AIDS are at increased risk for severe dengue due to their impaired immune systems. The condition can advance swiftly, and coinfections can further complicate therapy.

Cancer Patients: Individuals undergoing cancer treatment, such as chemotherapy, have decreased immune responses. Dengue infection in these patients requires careful management to prevent severe results.

Transplant Recipients: Organ transplant recipients on immunosuppressive medication are prone to dengue fever. Their immune deficiency makes them susceptible to serious diseases and consequences.

Management Strategies:

Tailored Treatment: Treatment strategies for people with comorbidities and immunocompromised patients must be individualized to address their specific needs and hazards. Close monitoring and modifications in therapy are essential.

Preventive Measures: Preventive methods, including vaccination (where appropriate), use of mosquito repellents, and environmental control measures, are crucial to minimizing the risk of dengue infection in these populations.

Integrated Care: A multidisciplinary strategy comprising infectious disease specialists, primary care doctors, and specialists in the management of comorbid illnesses is important to provide comprehensive care. Dengue fever provides considerable hurdles for susceptible populations, including children, pregnant women, elderly persons, those with comorbidities, and immunocompromised patients.

Tailored approaches in prevention, diagnosis, and management are necessary to protect and support these groups effectively.

Understanding the unique risks and requirements of these populations will assist healthcare providers in giving better care and improving outcomes for individuals most at risk of severe dengue illness. By focusing on tailored care and prevention techniques, we can lessen the impact of dengue fever and safeguard the health of susceptible individuals.

Chapter 10

Dengue Fever Vaccines and Medications

Dengue fever is a severe public health alarm in tropical and subtropical locations worldwide. Addressing this dilemma requires a comprehensive approach that includes vaccines, treatments, novel vector control measures, and joint initiatives. This section discusses the present status of dengue vaccines and treatments, innovative techniques for controlling the mosquito vector, and the importance of worldwide cooperation in treating this disease.

Available Vaccines and Their Efficacy

The development of vaccinations for dengue fever has been a complicated process due to the virus's unique properties and the presence of four distinct serotypes (DENV-1, DENV-2, DENV-3, and DENV-4). A good dengue vaccine must give immunity against all four serotypes to prevent severe illness and sequelae.

Dengvaxia (CYD-TDV):

Description: Dengvaxia, created by Sanofi Pasteur, is the first dengue vaccine to be licensed for use. It is a live attenuated vaccination designed to protect against all four dengue virus serotypes.

Efficacy: Clinical investigations have revealed that Dengvaxia gives moderate protection against dengue fever. Its efficiency varies by serotype and the individual's past exposure to dengue. The vaccination is more effective in persons who have had prior dengue illnesses.

Target Population: The World Health Organization (WHO) recommends Dengvaxia for individuals aged 9-45 years living in endemic areas with a high incidence of dengue. It is particularly indicated for those with a confirmed previous dengue infection, as the vaccine can raise the risk of severe dengue in seronegative persons (those who have never been infected previously).

TAK-003 (Dengue Vaccine Candidate):

Description: TAK-003, produced by Takeda Pharmaceutical Company, is alternative potential dengue vaccine candidate. It is a tetravalent live-attenuated vaccine addressing all four serotypes.

Efficacy: Phase III clinical trials have revealed that TAK-003 gives considerable protection against dengue illness. The vaccination has shown efficacy in both seropositive and seronegative persons, giving it a versatile alternative for varied groups.

Status: TAK-003 has completed its clinical trials and is pending regulatory approval in various countries. It has the potential to become a crucial tool in the fight against dengue once it achieves general authorization.

Other Vaccine Candidates:

DENVax: This vaccine candidate is been developed by Inviragen (now part of Takeda), uses a recombinant dengue virus to promote immunity against all four serotypes. Early clinical trials have shown promising outcomes.

Butantan-DV: Developed by the Butantan Institute in Brazil, this vaccine candidate is based on an attenuated dengue virus. Clinical trials are going to examine its safety and efficacy.

Novel Approaches for Vector Control

Controlling the Aedes mosquitoes that transmit dengue is a major component of dengue prevention. Traditional measures, such as pesticide spraying and reducing standing water, remain necessary but face problems due to mosquito resistance and environmental concerns. Novel approaches help to boost vector control efforts and reduce the spread of dengue.

Wolbachia-infected Mosquitoes:

Description: Wolbachia is a naturally occurring bacterium that can infect Aedes mosquitoes, limiting their ability to spread the dengue virus. When

Wolbachia-infected mosquitoes breed with wild mosquitoes, the germs propagate through the mosquito population.

Efficacy: Field investigations have demonstrated that releasing Wolbachia-infected mosquitoes into the environment can drastically reduce dengue transmission. The microorganisms limit epidemiologic replication within the mosquito, decreasing the possibility of the mosquito spreading the virus to people.

Implementation: Countries like Australia, Indonesia, and Brazil have launched Wolbachia-based vector control programs with encouraging results. This technology offers a sustainable and environmentally beneficial alternative to chemical insecticides.

Genetically Modified Mosquitoes:

Description: Genetic engineering techniques have been applied to develop Aedes mosquitoes with changes that either suppress their numbers or render them incapable of spreading dengue. One strategy includes releasing male mosquitoes with a gene that causes their offspring to die before reaching adulthood.

Efficacy: Trials have shown that releasing genetically modified mosquitoes can lead to a large reduction in local mosquito populations. This method has the potential to cut dengue transmission rates dramatically.

Challenges: Regulatory and ethical constraints, coupled with public acceptance, are essential aspects of the deployment of genetically modified mosquitoes. Ongoing research strives to solve these problems and optimize the effectiveness of this method.

Sterile Insect Technique (SIT):

Description: SIT includes releasing vast numbers of sterile male mosquitoes into the environment. When these guys mate with wild females, the resulting eggs do not hatch, leading to a reduction in the mosquito population.

Efficacy: SIT has been effectively used to control other insect pests and is currently being modified for Aedes mosquitoes. Field trials have demonstrated that SIT can reduce mosquito populations and minimize the risk of dengue transmission.

Implementation: Pilot programs in countries like China and Brazil have proved the feasibility of SIT for dengue vector control. Scaling up these initiatives could provide an extra instrument in the fight against dengue.

Collaborative Efforts in Combating Dengue

Dengue fever is a worldwide health concern that demands coordinated actions across governments and regions. Collaborative initiatives are needed to exchange knowledge, resources, and methods to effectively battle dengue. International organizations, governments, and research institutions play significant roles in these initiatives.

World Health Organization (WHO):

Role: The WHO provides leadership and coordination in the global response to dengue. It establishes standards, funds research, and enables information exchange across countries.

Initiatives: WHO's Global Strategy for Dengue Prevention and Control aims to minimize dengue morbidity and mortality through integrated vector management, improved diagnostics, and upgraded surveillance systems.

International Research Collaborations:

Partnerships: Collaborative research endeavors bring together scientists, healthcare workers, and public health specialists from around the world. These agreements promote the development of new vaccinations, diagnostic tools, and vector control approaches.

Projects: Examples of worldwide research collaborations are the European Union's DengueTools initiative and the Asia-Pacific Dengue Prevention Partnership. These programs focus on increasing dengue research and implementing evidence-based therapies.

Government and Non-Governmental Organizations (NGOs):

Government Programs: National governments in dengue-endemic nations execute vector control programs, vaccine campaigns, and public health education activities. These activities are generally sponsored by international money and technical expertise.

NGO Involvement: NGOs play a critical role in community participation, education, and advocacy. Organizations like the International Federation of Red Cross and Red Crescent Societies (IFRC) operate on the ground to raise awareness and advocate preventive measures.

Emerging Medications and Therapies

The fight against dengue fever has mostly centered on preventive and symptomatic treatment, as there is no specific antiviral medication currently available for dengue. However, current developments in research are paving the way for the creation of new drugs and therapies. These developing medicines aim to target the virus directly, ease symptoms more effectively, and prevent serious repercussions.

Antiviral Medications

One of the interesting areas of research is the development of antiviral medicines especially targeting the dengue virus. Antiviral drugs act by decreasing the virus's capacity to replicate, hence reducing the viral load and severity of the illness.

Favipiravir:

Description: Favipiravir is an antiviral medicine first developed to treat influenza. It has shown broad-spectrum effectiveness against different RNA viruses, including dengue.

Efficacy: Preclinical investigations and early-phase clinical trials have revealed that favipiravir can decrease dengue virus replication. Further research is needed to verify its safety and efficacy in treating dengue in humans.

Balapiravir:

Description: Balapiravir is another antiviral candidate that has shown potential in preclinical investigations. It targets the viral RNA polymerase, an enzyme important for viral replication.

Efficacy: While initial trials were not definitive, ongoing research intends to optimize its use and evaluate its usefulness in combination with other treatments.

Celgosivir:

Description: Celgosivir is an alpha-glucosidase inhibitor that has shown potential in suppressing the dengue virus in experimental settings.

Efficacy: Early trials indicate that celgosivir may reduce viral load and improve clinical outcomes. More thorough clinical trials are necessary to confirm these findings and define effective dose regimens.

Immunotherapies

Immunotherapy techniques are being researched to increase the body's immune response to dengue virus infection. These therapies try to improve the natural immune defenses and minimize the severity of the disease.

Monoclonal Antibodies:

Description: Monoclonal antibodies are laboratory-produced molecules designed to mimic the immune system's ability to fight off infections. They can be designed to target specific proteins on the surface of the dengue virus.

Efficacy: Several monoclonal antibodies have shown potential in neutralizing the dengue virus in preclinical investigations. Clinical trials are undertaken to test their safety and efficacy in humans.

Interferon-Based Therapies:

Description: Interferons are proteins formed by the immune system in response to viral infections. Interferon-based medicines aim to increase the body's antiviral response.

Efficacy: Some studies have suggested that interferon treatment can reduce dengue virus replication and improve clinical outcomes. Further study is needed to discover the appropriate time and dosage of interferon-based therapy.

Innovative Approaches and Technologies

Advancements in science and technology are creating new and novel techniques to tackle dengue disease. These include genetic modification, nanotechnology, artificial intelligence, and data analytics, all of which provide unique methods for dengue control and prevention.

Genetic Modification and Nanotechnology

Genetic Modification of Mosquitoes:

Description: Genetic modification techniques are being utilized to alter the genetic makeup of Aedes mosquitoes, the principal carriers of dengue. These alterations can render mosquito's incapable of transmitting the virus or diminish their population.

Sterile Insect Technique (SIT): This includes releasing genetically sterile male mosquitoes into the environment. When these guys mate with wild females, the resulting eggs do not hatch, leading to a reduction in the mosquito population.

Gene Drive Technology: Gene drive systems promote the inheritance of specific genes to rapidly propagate alterations among wild mosquito populations. This is used to lower mosquito fertility or boost resistance to dengue virus.

Nanotechnology:

Description: Nanotechnology is the manipulation of matter on an atomic or molecular scale to develop new materials and gadgets with unique properties. In the context of dengue, nanotechnology can be employed to produce targeted medicine delivery systems and diagnostic instruments.

Nanoparticle-Based Vaccines: Researchers are studying the use of nanoparticles to generate more effective dengue vaccines. These nanoparticles can improve the immune response and give longer-lasting protection.

Drug Delivery Systems: Nanoparticles can be tailored to carry antiviral medications directly to infected cells, boosting the efficacy of the treatment while limiting side effects.

Artificial Intelligence and Data Analytics in Dengue Control

Artificial intelligence (AI) and data analytics are transforming the way we analyze and control dengue disease. These technologies offer more precise predictions, effective resource allocation, and focused actions.

Predictive Modeling:

Description: AI systems can evaluate enormous volumes of data to anticipate dengue outbreaks with great accuracy. These models take into account elements such as weather patterns, mosquito population dynamics, and human movement.

Efficacy: Predictive modeling assists public health authorities in implementing preventative measures in a timely way, decreasing the effect of dengue outbreaks. It enables the strategic allocation of resources and targeted vector control activities.

Surveillance Systems:

Description: Advanced surveillance systems use AI and machine learning to monitor and analyze data from numerous sources, including hospital records, social media, and environmental sensors.

Efficacy: These technologies provide real-time insights into dengue transmission patterns, helping to identify hotspots and emerging trends. They boost the ability to respond promptly to outbreaks and conduct control measures successfully.

Personalized Medicine:

Description: AI can be used to produce personalized treatment recommendations based on an individual's genetic makeup and disease profile. This method tries to optimize treatment outcomes and limit the risk of serious consequences.

Efficacy: Personalized medicine has the potential to improve patient outcomes by adapting therapies to the specific needs of each individual. It signifies a shift towards more accurate and effective healthcare.

Public Health Campaigns:

Description: Data analytics can be used to create and conduct more successful public health programs. By examining data on human behavior, communication patterns, and community engagement, public health authorities can build targeted treatments that resonate with certain communities.

Efficacy: Targeted public health initiatives are more likely to accomplish targeted results, such as improved knowledge of preventive measures and higher vaccination rates. They make sure that resources are used efficiently and effectively.

The fight against dengue fever is evolving swiftly with the arrival of new treatments, novel technologies, and superior data analytics. Antiviral drugs, immunotherapies, genetic manipulation, nanotechnology, artificial intelligence, and data analytics are revolutionizing the landscape of dengue control and prevention. These advancements give new hope for lowering the incidence of dengue disease and protecting vulnerable communities worldwide. Collaborative efforts among scientists, healthcare professionals, governments, and communities are necessary to utilize these advances and make sustainable progress in the fight against dengue. Through ongoing study, innovation, and cooperation, we may move towards a future where dengue fever is effectively controlled and its impact on public health is minimized.

The fight against dengue fever is a monument to the intricacy of global health concerns. With its extensive prevalence in tropical and subtropical countries, dengue fever constitutes a substantial hazard to public health worldwide. This thorough resource has covered numerous parts of dengue fever, from its biological underpinnings and transmission dynamics to diagnostic procedures, treatment options, and preventative initiatives. As we finish this debate, it is vital to consolidate the key ideas, underline the importance of ongoing education and awareness, assess the future prognosis for dengue prevention and treatment, and reflect on the necessity of continued research and global collaboration.

Recap of Key Points

Dengue fever is a mosquito-borne epidemiologic disease caused by four distinct serotypes of the dengue virus (DENV-1 to DENV-4). It is transmitted predominantly by Aedes mosquitoes, particularly Aedes aegypti and Aedes albopictus. The disease displays in a ranging from mild dengue fever to severe forms such as dengue hemorrhagic fever (DHF) and dengue shock syndrome (DSS). Key symptoms include high temperature, severe headache, pain behind the eyes, joint and muscular pain, rash, and moderate bleeding signs. Severe cases can lead to serious problems, including plasma leakage, hemorrhage, and organ dysfunction, which require rapid medical attention and careful care.

Diagnostic procedures for dengue fever include the identification of the NS1 antigen, IgM/IgG antibodies, and viral RNA using polymerase chain reaction (PCR). Differential diagnosis is crucial to separate dengue from other febrile infections such as malaria, chikungunya, and Zika virus infection. Effective management of dengue entails supportive care, including fluid replacement, pain medication, and constant monitoring for complications. For severe cases, guidelines emphasize the significance of immediate hospitalization, proper fluid management, and watchful monitoring for indicators of shock and bleeding.

Preventing dengue disease rests on vector control techniques and personal protective strategies. Eliminating mosquito breeding areas, utilizing insect repellents, wearing protective clothes, and conducting community-based activities are critical components of dengue prevention. The discovery and distribution of vaccinations, such as Dengvaxia, constitute a significant advancement, however, their usage is subject to particular guidelines and limitations based on serostatus and age.

Importance of Ongoing Education and Awareness

Education and awareness are crucial to controlling dengue illness. Public understanding of the disease, its transmission, symptoms, and prevention methods is vital for minimizing the incidence and effect of dengue. Awareness campaigns should target multiple audiences, including individuals, communities, healthcare professionals, and policymakers.

For individuals and groups, education should emphasize the necessity of reducing mosquito breeding areas, recognizing early symptoms, obtaining appropriate medical assistance, and sticking to preventive measures. Schools, workplaces, and community centers can serve as useful platforms for disseminating information and generating community engagement in dengue-preventive activities.

Healthcare workers have a critical role in the early detection and management of dengue patients. Continued medical education and training programs should equip healthcare providers with the information and abilities to diagnose, treat, and manage dengue fever efficiently. This includes remaining educated about the newest guidelines, developments in diagnostic methods, and novel treatments.

Policymakers and public health authorities must prioritize dengue management in their agendas, allocating funding for vector control programs, research initiatives, and healthcare facilities. International cooperation and collaboration are required to address the transnational nature of dengue and execute coordinated policies for prevention and control.

Future Outlook for Dengue Prevention and Treatment

The future of dengue prevention and treatment holds promise, driven by breakthroughs in science, technology, and global health initiatives. Several locations are ready to make important contributions to the fight against dengue.

Vaccine Development: Ongoing research aims to generate more effective and broadly protective dengue vaccinations. Current vaccinations, such as Dengvaxia, have certain restrictions and are indicated exclusively for those with past dengue illness. Future vaccines should ideally produce long-lasting immunity against all four dengue virus serotypes, be safe for all age groups, and be accessible in endemic places.

Antiviral Therapies: The development of specialized antiviral drugs for dengue is a critical field of research. Promising candidates, including favipiravir, favipiravir, and celgosivir, are undergoing clinical testing. These medications try to suppress viral replication and lower the severity of infection. Successful antiviral medicines would mark a substantial breakthrough in the clinical management of dengue illness.

Unique Vector Control: Advances in genetic modification and nanotechnology offer unique ways to vector control. Techniques such as the Sterile Insect Technique (SIT) and gene drive technologies can lower mosquito populations or render them incapable of transmitting the virus. Nanotechnology can strengthen diagnostic tools and produce targeted medication delivery systems, boosting the efficacy of therapies.

Artificial Intelligence and Data Analytics: Artificial intelligence (AI) and data analytics are changing dengue surveillance and response tactics. Predictive modeling, enhanced monitoring systems, and customized medicine approaches can promote early detection, resource allocation, and focused therapies. AI-driven public health campaigns can boost knowledge and compliance with preventive measures, thereby reducing the burden of dengue.

Final Thoughts on the Importance of Continued Research and Global Collaboration

The fight against dengue fever is far from ending, and continuing research and global collaboration are vital to ensure sustained progress. Scientific research is the basis of generating new therapies, vaccines, and diagnostic tools. It is crucial to encourage and fund research programs that explore novel approaches to dengue prevention and control.

Global collaboration is vital in tackling the transnational aspect of dengue and exchanging knowledge, resources, and best practices. International organizations, governments, non-governmental organizations, and the corporate sector must work together to implement coordinated plans, strengthen healthcare systems, and expand access to preventative measures and treatments.

Public health strategies should stress community engagement and participation, acknowledging the essential role of individuals and communities in dengue prevention. Empowering communities via information, resources, and assistance can develop resilience and lessen the effects of dengue outbreaks.

The fight against dengue fever demands a broad approach, combining scientific innovation, effective public health policies, and worldwide cooperation. By remaining informed, supporting research, and working together, we can make great gains in lowering the incidence of dengue fever and protecting vulnerable communities globally. Through continuous efforts, we may picture a world where dengue is no longer a major public health hazard, and communities can prosper free from the fear and effect of this crippling disease.